A SURVIVOR'S GUIDE TO
KICKING
CANCER'S ASS

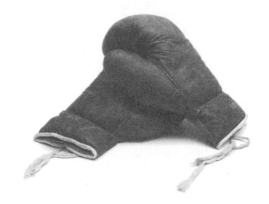

Dena Mendes

HAY
HOUSE

HAY HOUSE, INC.
Carlsbad, California • New York City
London • Sydney • Johannesburg
Vancouver • Hong Kong • New Delhi

Published and distributed in the United States by: Hay House, Inc.:
www.hayhouse.com • *Published and distributed in Australia by:* Hay
House Australia Pty. Ltd.: www.hayhouse.com.au • *Published and
distributed in the United Kingdom by:* Hay House UK, Ltd.: www.
hayhouse.co.uk • *Published and distributed in the Republic of South
Africa by:* Hay House SA (Pty), Ltd.: www.hayhouse.co.za • *Distributed
in Canada by:* Raincoast: www.raincoast.com • *Published in India by:*
Hay House Publishers India: www.hayhouse.co.in

Cover design: Christy Salinas • *Interior design:* Pam Homan

The author of this book does not dispense medical advice or pre-
scribe the use of any technique as a form of treatment for physical, emotional, or medical problems without the advice of a physician, either
directly or indirectly. The intent of the author is only to offer information of a general nature to help you in your quest for emotional and
spiritual well-being. In the event you use any of the information in this
book for yourself, which is your constitutional right, the author and the
publisher assume no responsibility for your actions.

Library of Congress Cataloging-in-Publication Data

Mendes, Dena.
A survivor's guide to kicking cancer's ass / Dena Mendes.
p. cm.
ISBN 978-1-4019-3154-4 (pbk.)
1. Cancer--Popular works. 2. Cancer--Patients--Popular works. I. Title.
RC263.M42 2011
616.99'4--dc23
2011024043

ISBN: 978-1-4019-3154-4
Digital ISBN: 978-1-4019-3155-1

14 13 12 11 4 3 2 1
1st edition, November 2011

Printed in the United States of America

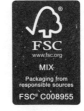

*I dedicate this book to my children,
the love and light of my life . . .
and who stuck by me through it all!*

*I dedicate this book to people of every
age who have endured the challenges
of turning chaos into opportunity,
nightmares into dreams.*

*I dedicate this book to people who
have had to turn themselves inside out
through horrific amounts of pain,
the kind of catastrophic life-changing events
that would crumble buildings.*

*To all the fighters, to all the survivors,
and to those who continue to fight each day.
To the ones who have lost love,
lost limbs, lost faith or hope.
To those who have lost their lives
like my sweet brother, Bradley . . .*

I dedicate this book to you.

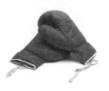

CONTENTS

INTRODUCTION

The Rabbit Hole

"I wonder if I've been changed in the night? Let me think: was I the same when I got up this morning? I almost think I can remember feeling a little different. But if I'm not the same, the next question is, Who in the world am I? Ah, <u>that's</u> the great puzzle!"

— FROM *ALICE'S ADVENTURES IN WONDERLAND*,
BY LEWIS CARROLL

Whenever I'm asked to describe what being diagnosed with cancer is like, what instantly floods my mind are images of a surreal and absurdist musical being acted out on some stage. It's impossible to expect the human brain to grasp the paralyzing devastation that comes from that single word: *cancer*. I liken it to Alice's first trip down the rabbit hole, as she lost her footing and her world spun out of control. Just like Alice, I was catapulted into a bizarre misadventure that ultimately resulted in a beautiful metamorphosis.

Before I was diagnosed with cancer, I was finally having the wonderful life I'd always dreamed of after a childhood filled with abuse. The experiences I went through as a young girl were traumatic, yet I believed they were normal.

"Children should be seen and not heard" was my father's credo, and we marched to the beat of his drum or else we paid dearly. My mother was too young and self-absorbed to be a mother. My parents' inability to be attentive, compassionate, and loving was not their fault, as they were products of their own environment. Yet the more I craved the love and attention that I couldn't get, the angrier and more rebellious I became. I believe I was suffering from depression and low self-esteem, and I continued on this path for years.

I often became ill from physical and emotional abuse as well as the typical teenage poor-quality diet, made up of chemical-laden, processed foods. When I was 17, I developed a spastic colon (also known as "irritable bowel syndrome") and colitis. During this time, I had the privilege of stumbling across my first guru, Max Vanorman, who literally saved my life. He taught me to turn the damage from my family dysfunction into a desire to learn more about mental and emotional healing—and he was the first person who ever showed me the connection between food and how we feel and function physically, mentally, and emotionally. Thanks to Max, I not only healed from my stomach issues within three weeks, I was also inspired to study natural healing in all its capacities.

I went on to attend Arizona State University, studying communications, broadcast journalism, and public health. I wanted to combine my interest in natural modalities with the ability to "share the health." While earning my bachelor of arts degree, I worked as a research reporter and medical-news reporting assistant for NBC KPNX-TV 12 in Phoenix. Even back then, I tried to squeeze my "natural stories" in between sports and what I considered fluff—but in the late '80s, people had never heard of fish oil or probiotics, so my stories weren't well received.

After leaving Arizona, I moved to Chicago, where I met my husband, Steve. At first his friends and family thought I was strange, since I introduced them to natural remedies labeled with bizarre names such as "wormwood" and "bladder wrack." Steve had two great boys from a previous marriage, August and Brice; he and I then had the first girl in the family, Paris, and soon after came our son Jet. Once I had children, I felt lucky to spend my days caring for and nurturing them. I was happy and fulfilled . . . until the first bolt of lightning hit our household in 1998.

Steve was diagnosed with bile-duct cancer, a typically terminal form of the disease. It was my first serious call to action. I quickly assembled the troops and worked around the clock to heal him. I voraciously devoured everything I could learn about cancer so I could help save my husband's life. Due to all the medical and natural tools we were blessed with, as well as his own amazing sense of fortitude, he survived, and he's healthy today.

Unfortunately, there was no rest for the weary. Less than two years later, a second bolt of lightning struck— and this time, it hit *me*. My "cancer career" began when my gynecologist suggested, "Let's watch this mass in your breast." I had a scar in my right breast that had formed years earlier when I accidentally slammed it in a car door (ouch), and after keeping an eye on it for some time, it became clear to him that the scar or mass in my right breast had become rounder and more defined.

I felt that mammograms emitted too much radiation, so I went for a thermograph, which is an imaging technique that uses infrared sensors to map differences in heat levels across your breasts. According to the report, I had no signs of cancer.

After another year of watching the mass in my breast with thermographs, I finally broke down at my gynecologist's insistence and went for a regular mammogram with a specialist.

I got the call the following morning, and I couldn't believe the news. This specialist, whom I didn't even know, was hysterical as he told me I had what "looked like cancer," and that I "must have an immediate lumpectomy or suffer the consequences." It reminded me of the childhood story *Chicken Little,* when he frantically cried, "The sky is falling! The sky is falling!" (When it comes to cancer, there's more drama than a soap opera.) After I hung up with the specialist, I called my husband in tears. I thought for sure I was dying.

I made an appointment at a local hospital, yet when I met the surgeon who was to perform the lumpectomy, he seemed so cold and distant that I instantly knew I didn't like him. So why did I let him operate on me? Frankly, I didn't know I had a choice. I was so scared that I simply did whatever "the expert" told me to do.

After the lumpectomy, I patiently waited for the results, suffering on pins and needles, like all good patients do. Certainly I didn't want to seem too demanding—who was I to demand anything? By week four, the call finally came. It was the surgeon, saying what sounded like, "Blah blah blah . . . I didn't get it all . . . blah blah blah . . . you're screwed . . . blah blah blah."

In other words, what he was really explaining, in all his medical mumbo jumbo, was that he had not removed the entire pea-sized tumor—the biopsy had revealed "dirty margins." You see, when surgeons remove a tumor, they also remove some of the tissue that surrounds it; this tissue is called the "surgical margins." A pathologist will later examine these margins to determine whether the cancer has spread. If they don't find cancer cells in it, then you have "clean" (or "negative") margins. If they *do* find cancer cells, then you have "dirty" (or "positive") margins, and that means you also still have cancer cells in your body.

Calling me four weeks later was far too late for this surgeon to let me know that he had just released the hounds of hell into my body. I came to find out later that I originally had DCIS, or ductal carcinoma in situ. A *ductal carcinoma* is a cancer within the milk duct, and *in situ* means that the cancer was totally contained and noninvasive. In layman's terms, this means I had a totally encapsulated tumor that, when removed properly, would have had an extremely low chance of ever rearing its ugly head again, especially for someone like me, who practiced such a healthy lifestyle.

I was supposed to respect this doctor for having some initials after his name, but I felt like he'd just signed initials after *my* name. They read: "DOA" (that is, Dead on Arrival).

So began the fight for my life. This was the pivotal moment when I decided that no matter what happened next, I would empower myself and be prepared to kick some ass.

I turned to my close friend Dr. Merrick Ross, for the distinct privilege of cleaning up the last surgeon's mess. Yet since it was Christmastime, he couldn't see me for another three weeks. It would be a total of seven weeks from the time of the lumpectomy until my appointment at MD Anderson Cancer Center in Houston with Dr. Ross. Seven weeks for the lingering cancer cells to percolate and roam freely throughout my body. Even so, after the cleanup surgery, Dr. Ross called with the good news. I had clean margins . . . they got it all. Yeah!

That was it. I was done. Or so I thought. Three months later, I had a pea-size lump pop out in my breast directly above the scar site from the lumpectomy. I found myself back at MD Anderson, where they told me the cancer had spread to the internal mammary sentinel node, the main lymph node within my breast. This is rare, as cancer typically spreads to the axillary lymph nodes, which are located in the armpit.

Dr. Ross conducted a lymph-node dissection, which was the most devastating of all the surgeries I would eventually have. When I awoke, I found out that I had to have four rounds of chemotherapy. I cried as I remembered all the pain and suffering my husband had gone through four years earlier with his cancer. Watching him undergo chemo was so painful that when faced with it myself, I wasn't sure I could endure it.

I came home to meet with an oncologist, whom I didn't like. She was worse than cold—she was placating *and* cold. She never once told me that the chemotherapy they were about to give me wasn't the correct regimen. The cancer I had was 100 percent HER2/neu positive, and the chemo they were about to administer to me was designed for estrogen-dominant tumors. They had nothing else to offer; it simply was the "standard of care" available at that time. In fact, instead of telling me the truth and letting me decide whether I wanted this harsh treatment that was not conclusively effective on HER2/neu tumors, the doctors and nurses kept robotically repeating, "It's the standard of care." I didn't even know what that meant.

Six months later, the toxic overload left me a depleted and ravaged 90-pound rag doll. To add insult to injury, after a routine mammogram a year later, I learned that the chemotherapy had not worked to kill the cancer. It had actually weakened my immune system when I needed it most. The films showed that microcalcifications, which look like grains of salt but are actually tiny groups of calcium deposits, had filled my breast. This signaled that something was wrong. I knew I wanted to remove my breast as soon as I could—whether it was cancerous or not.

In my weakened state, I stupidly let the doctors conduct a needle biopsy to make sure the microcalcifications hadn't escaped the breast area. Although the mammogram films had showed that the cancer appeared to be totally encapsulated, they still wanted to have a poking party. When I think of this scene today, it conjures up visions of mad scientists whirling around with giant syringes. I remember the immediate bad feeling I had, and that I wanted to stop them but wasn't sure how.

For this procedure—known as a stereotactic (or mammographically guided) breast biopsy—I was asked to lie down on a table, complete with a hole to drop my breast through. And then, from under the table, a machine with an automatic, spring-loaded needle was placed up against my breast to biopsy. No more degrading machine exists. Anyway, the results confirmed what we suspected: the microcalcifications were cancerous but contained to the breast.

Weeks later (once again, after Christmas break), I showed up for my scheduled mastectomy. The removal part wasn't so bad. What was disturbing was the call I received three weeks later. It wasn't the news I had hoped. The pathology report from the mastectomy said I now had a "microscopic invasion." This meant that some microscopic amounts of cancer cells had escaped the breast and were set free to roam anywhere they pleased in my body. Like a game of hide-and-seek, these tiny cancer cells could hide for years. Although the doctor told me I was technically free of the disease after the mastectomy, he sounded a bit nervous about my future due to this invasion.

My intuition is typically correct. When the doctor read the pathology report to me, I remember instantly thinking, *I screwed up when I let them poke needles in my breast.* For the next four years, I would lie awake in bed with Paris, my precious little girl; and Jet, my funny little boy; and I'd start to tear up as I inhaled their sweet, innocent smell. I knew in my soul that I wasn't finished yet, but I wondered, *Will I see them graduate? Will I see them get married? Will I see my grandchildren?*

Even so, I was determined to stay positive and to be proactive. I began my mission to revive myself through natural modalities, alternative remedies, physical conditioning, and emotional healing. I realized that I needed to find a doctor who would be open to traditional *and* alternative health care, one who would be honest and honor me as an intelligent human being.

I knew I had to stay in fighting shape. I relied on my healthy lifestyle by using nutritious food as my first line of defense. I also continued to see a bevy of natural healers— including naturopaths, acupuncturists, and herbalists— who worked with me to create and implement a master plan to keep my immune system at peak performance. I felt strong . . . but I also couldn't help feeling like a sitting duck.

I decided to have my mastectomy breast redone due to the pain I was experiencing from the staples that had been used to hold the implant in place originally. I never imagined that replacing it could be so difficult. The reason I'm sharing this is to further drive home my point about being very clear in your communications with doctors, nurses, and anesthesiologists. They are busy professionals who are, I'm sure, doing the best they can. With that being said, they see many patients a day and are often overworked and overtired. Don't expect them to remember what you need or even guess. For example, I chose the implant I wanted with the doctor, but he must have forgotten by the time I got into surgery. I also explained my delicate condition to anesthesiology; they must have forgotten as well. They administered enough drugs for a 200-pound man instead of for my 115-pound frame.

One week later, I had to go for another surgery because they put in the wrong implant. These two surgeries back-to-back took their toll on me physically. When I awoke, my kidneys were completely depleted. The pain was beyond comprehension; I thought I was dying. My macrobiotic friend came to my rescue with compresses of ginger and daikon radish (boiled together and then soaked in cloths), which she placed directly on my kidneys. What a huge help!

I have always questioned if my next recurrence was brought on by the stress of this surgical nightmare— although I'm sure it was only a matter of time. Whatever the case, the cancer was back. This time it wasn't confined to the breast; it had metastasized (spread) to my bones, lungs, and neck. Although I'd been expecting this news,

I wasn't prepared for the extent of it. Even if you have an intuitive knowing and have heard the words before, you can never truly prepare yourself for the phrase "You have cancer." These are the most frightening, surreal, and life-changing words you will ever hear.

At this point I was referred to the oncologist I am still with today: Dr. Douglas Merkel at Northwestern Memorial Hospital. I liked him right away because he was direct and didn't talk down to me as he offered the newest targeted drug therapy for HER2/neu called Herceptin. I did eight weeks of a chemo regimen called Vinorelbine, along with the Herceptin, and I kicked ass all the way through it. I remained on the Herceptin and went about my life.

Four years later, I was once again in the hot seat of emotional and physical stress. It was so intense that I was having seizures and didn't know it. I kept dropping things; I couldn't type with my left hand; I felt dizzy and off balance. One week later, I had a massive seizure due to a right-lobe brain tumor. What I found out later is that Herceptin cannot cross the blood-brain barrier, meaning that it cannot protect the brain from metastasis. I was rushed to Evanston Hospital to undergo brain surgery with the very well-known neurosurgeon Dr. Ivan Ciric. He is the most brilliant man I have ever met. I felt so safe with him; he made absolutely sure there would be no lingering cancer cells by removing a thick surgical margin around the tumor to ensure it was clean. This was like an insurance policy against a recurrence.

The day after an eight-hour surgery, I was lured outside by the power of the sun. I strolled out of ICU, IV pole in tow, and right there on the crisp green lawn, I enjoyed my own private yoga session. I am typically Trouble with a capital T, so it was no surprise when the hospital staff nicely suggested that I leave after two days instead of the usual four-day stay.

●○●

Like Alice, I too have grown since I started that trip down the rabbit hole. When I first heard the word *cancer*, I was blown away. I couldn't string a simple sentence together, and that's saying a lot for someone who talks as much as I do. Of course, I questioned how this could happen to me. Now, all these years later, I realize there is so much more to cancer than just the physicality of it.

I've grown, learned, and have had a complete metamorphosis. I've gone through dozens of tests, treatments, and surgeries; and I celebrate my uniqueness by discovering what my body, mind, and spirit need for me to kick this disease's ass. After my first few diagnoses, it got to the point that I'd actually laugh and say, "Don't worry, there are no problems—there are only solutions. We shall figure this out together." The doctors used to look at me like I was crazy. After working with me for a while, they realized that I'm simply empowered.

My diagnosis is not who I am, it is only what has happened to me. The real story began *after* I was diagnosed. What's far more important is what I plan to do in the future. I hate to use such a trite saying as "Cancer is a gift," but it truly is for people who are willing to look directly into the eye of the storm, wake up, and turn themselves inside out to all the possibilities. The new you is the gift.

The gift cancer gave *me* was that nothing would ever be scary again. Through it all, I learned to face my greatest fear of all: the fear of failure. I went on to pursue every impossible possibility, and then watch as each dream came true, one by one. For example, I wrote books for children; a natural-foods cookbook; and a theatrical musical about cancer, *Standard of Care*. My dear friend Claudia Lubin and I created an in-school program called "the Food Detectives." We taught kids how to empower themselves by reading labels, becoming more self-aware, and making healthy lifestyle choices.

I took another step toward realizing my dreams when I enrolled in a yoga teacher–training program. During the course of training, I went through a mastectomy, contracted pneumonia, and experienced the death of my brother (who was also my best friend). I kept going, though. I will never forget the closing ceremony—I couldn't stop crying because it felt so good to work so hard and accomplish something for myself.

A few years ago, I developed a program and website called "Dena's Healthy U" (**www.denashealthyu.com**), a venue whereby I "share the health" with others. In addition, I earned a doctorate in naturopathy. Yet more important than these credentials is the sheer amount of self-awareness and intuitive prowess I've gained over the years, to heal myself and others. And that brings us to this book.

I've written it to be of service to those who seek to find the balance between strength and surrender, the fighter and the graceful dancer, the poet and the warrior. I have unveiled the mystery of traditional medical protocols while combining the power of implementing healing foods, guides and gurus, elixirs and remedies, and all manner of alternative-healing modalities to empower you on your journey.

It is with all of my vast culled knowledge, gained over the past two decades, that I offer you the material within these pages—where you will find wisdom, humor, insight, and personal anecdotes that will help you navigate through this, your very own beautiful health-awakening opportunity.

Although my diagnosis originated from the breast, I've created this book to assist in all cases of cancer. No matter if you're a man or woman, young or old; if you're undergoing traditional therapies or have just finished treatments of any kind; if you're battling the disease yourself or helping a loved one through it . . . this guide is for you.

A Survivor's Guide to Kicking Cancer's Ass will inspire you to take control of your health, to gain a new sense of yourself, to use your intuition, and to implement a wealth of healing options. On your journey, you'll discover remedies for different maladies that might come up along the way. You will become a self-health detective and follow your own intuition as you learn to mix and match remedies and modalities, in order to heal thyself.

Like Alice, you may ask the question, "Who in the world am I?" Keep in mind: your life is a journey that comprises assembling the pieces of your identity, fitting together your experiences, and having faith and trust in your path and yourself.

So, let's get started!

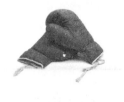

CHAPTER ONE

Diagnosis:
When the Shit Hits the Fan

If you're reading this book, then the shit has obviously hit the fan. You've been diagnosed with cancer, or you know someone who has. You're probably more than freaked out, and you have a million questions that you feel you need the answers to right away.

The most important thing you need to know is that it isn't as much about the "answers" as it is about the journey and the amazing health-awakening experience in store for you. It is time to reinvent yourself; that's what this means. Don't worry, you're not alone. I am here for you—as are so many others—to guide you through this painful, traumatic, confusing, enlightening, and beautiful transformation.

When I was diagnosed almost a decade ago, I was just as scared and confused as you are now. The perfect way to describe the feeling when you first hear the words "You have cancer" is that you're burning outside, like you're on fire—yet you're bitterly cold on the inside, sort of like a brain freeze after drinking a 7-Eleven Slurpee too fast. It is truly an out-of-body experience.

At first, I was afraid I was going to die. In fact, the fear was so paralyzing that I was ready to do whatever the doctors told me I needed to do to survive, no questions asked. I wish someone had been there to tell me to take a step back; take some time to absorb and process what I'd just been told; and come up with pertinent questions for the "all-knowing, all-seeing" beings we believe our doctors to be. We think that they are infallible and know everything. I'm here to tell you this: they *don't* know everything, so take your time and ask plenty of questions.

Being diagnosed truly does feel like "falling down the rabbit hole." It's a fantastical trip, that's for sure, so put on your seat belt and join me in this chance to turn yourself inside out, to dive directly into the present moment like a warrior. I have found that something this big doesn't just go away until it has taught us all we need to know. So bless it for coming to teach you. Then dig deep . . . but don't take it too seriously. Trust me, you will be opening to many new and exciting ideas, so have some fun with your awakening as you allow a whole new world to unfold, one that is rewarding and fulfilling beyond your wildest imagination.

Forget words like *hope,* which, I have come to learn, stems from a feeling of lack and fear. Reaching our breaking point or having the earth crumble beneath our feet is neither a punishment nor a sign that the end is near; it is, however, a sign of enlightenment. Create the gift by holding hands with your fear. Stay with your fear, get to know it—what does it smell like, feel like, look like? The key is to stop struggling against fear, because, like quicksand, the more you struggle, the faster you sink. Instead of numbing yourself with pills or a drink, let's dare to wake up and look directly at the scary monster.

Now that you know your fear intimately, you know that it can't kill you this minute. Welcome to my world—let's get to work and kick some ass. In this book, I proudly share all my resources, remedies, and protocols that helped me to not just survive, but thrive.

It seems that no matter what kind of cancer my clients are dealing with, the question is always the same: "Do you have some sort of guide to help me through this?" I've come up with just that—a step-by-step guide that serves as a life preserver for you and your loved ones.

Choosing Your Doctor

First and foremost, it is imperative that you find a physician who will be your partner and allow you to become an active participant in your healing process. As you conduct your search, here are some rules of thumb to follow:

- You must feel comfortable with the doctor you select, so search for someone who is warm instead of cold and callous. He or she should be patient and really listen to you when you ask questions or have requests, not rushing to get you out of the room.

- Your doctor should speak to you on an equal level so that you clearly understand what's being explained to you.

- Look for someone positive and not dramatic in nature. Remember, his or her attitude will affect your healing process and your outcome.

- Try to find a practitioner who offers you some alternative health-care modalities, literature on integrative therapies, and new protocols available. Ask if he or she is willing to give you a prescription for complementary health care, such as lymphatic drainage.

- Finally, be aware of your specific insurance plan and what it covers.

It's also extremely important that you follow your intuition. If your gut feeling about some medical professional leaves you unsure, uncomfortable, uncertain, and invalidated, find another one.

I remember when, early on in my journey, I met a doctor I instantly didn't like. I thought he was cold, impersonal, and impatient—but I stuck with him anyway. Why would I have done that? It is common for people to feel inferior to doctors' "brilliance," and to do whatever they say without question. But for me, it was also a gender thing. I was still stuck in the mind-set of a little girl who had an overbearing father. I was afraid to speak out of turn, let alone ask too many questions.

The doctor I ultimately chose to help me through my process is wonderful, open, patient, and understanding; and he didn't bully me by using fear tactics. He also allows me to create my own healing regimens outside of the hospital, such as combining natural healers, organic foods, alternative supplements, and other treatments.

Always keep this in mind: *Doctors work for you.* You pay them, and you have every right to demand what you want.

I am a total advocate for speaking your truth and expressing your expectations in a respectful way to doctors; they *are* human, after all, and should be informed if they're not satisfying your needs as a patient.

I once had a radiologist tell me that she was only allotted so many minutes with each patient, and it was very difficult for her to tell people they had cancer and then shove them out the door. Since hearing that, I remember to tell my doctors, "I won't be leaving until I'm done." Don't forget, you are paying for this appointment. You can sit on that table as long as you like until all questions are answered to your satisfaction.

Write It Down

Here's another great piece of advice: In the midst of chaos and stress, it can be difficult to stay focused, let alone remember anything. I suggest you write it down. Don't leave that examining room or let him run out until you're satisfied. Afterward, go home, think about what you were told, discuss it with other people, and get a second opinion—and then third and fourth opinions if you need them. But be careful. If you solicit five opinions, you'll get five different answers.

You may be afraid to make any kind of demands of your doctor, or to ask him to spend more time explaining something you don't understand, fearing that this would make you seem pushy or stupid. Yet I've seen firsthand how damaging these feelings can be.

Recently, I went to the hospital to visit a client who was suffering from lung cancer. She was a frail 84-year-old woman who hadn't eaten in two weeks and had dropped 15 pounds. I was blown away when her family told me they weren't allowed to change her diet because any and all natural foods were considered "food supplements" and should not be "taken," as if they were dangerous pharmaceuticals.

This poor woman and her family were at the mercy of her physician. They felt as if their hands were tied, so they did exactly what he told them to do. This wasn't necessary. I pointed out that I'd been through the same treatments as their mother, and that because of the tools I used to empower myself and rebuild my immune system, I looked and felt great. Still, the family was so concerned about offending the doctor that they looked like deer stuck in headlights.

In a weak and timid voice, my client told me, "We can't even get near the doctor—he doesn't want to listen to us." I was so shocked and angry that I felt like screaming at this man. All I could think was, *Really, who works for whom here? Do we live in that much fear of our doctors? Don't we pay an astronomical amount for their fees, services, and medications?*

Then I remembered how I felt at first. I also felt inferior to the "superior doctor." I didn't know that I had a choice or a voice. I didn't use mine in the beginning either, and it almost cost me my life. But I found that there was a better way, one that required a working relationship with my doctor based on mutual respect. Since then, I never go into any doctor's office without my trusty notebook and pen in hand. I've learned to write down my questions beforehand so I won't forget to ask a thing. Even if I feel that the doctor is trying to push me out of the room, I just smile and say, "I waited for over an hour to get into this little room, and now you're stuck with me until I'm satisfied."

So, take notes and ask your doctor to repeat his comments if necessary. He should slow down or explain concepts more thoroughly so you can better understand what's being said. Ask for a direct phone number or pager so you can call if you think of further questions after you leave, which you inevitably will. At the end, don't forget to smile sweetly and say, "Thank you so much for your time."

Be Strong

When people call me after a cancer diagnosis, I tell them with total confidence that when they're done crying, they will absolutely pick themselves up, dust themselves off, and live another day. I say that they get to become someone new, not only for themselves but also for their loved ones. The reasons these individuals have been diagnosed can be deep and vast. I assure them that they shouldn't worry about that now as the answers will present themselves soon enough. I had one client, for instance, who learned everything there was to know about alternative modalities so when the time came, she was instrumental in helping to heal her son when he went through a similar health crisis.

What is important for you to know right now is that you can live a long and healthy life. Many individuals live with cancer today just as people live with diabetes. Prepare yourself just as you would for a test in school. If you don't study, you will fail. So "know thy subject." Before gathering the tools you will need for this battle, you must quiet your mind. This might not make sense while you're in panic mode, but believe me, by the end of this book, it will. For now, suffice it to say that through stillness, the world will be unmasked and will freely offer you the intuitive answers you seek on your journey. You will first need to turn inward to the silence of your soul.

To do this, I suggest you set aside some time each day to sit comfortably in a special space with your spine erect. As you breathe, follow the exhale . . . every time you catch yourself thinking, simply say, "Thinking" and then let it go, like a cloud that floats away, effortlessly. Stay in this present state for a few moments at first; you'll see how the time expands with your mind. You'll find yourself craving this space where you can safely observe the chaos and fear, where you can listen to *you*.

Many people who call me feel as if they have been given a death sentence. When I tell them that it is entirely feasible for them to lead full, healthy, and long lives, I can actually hear them straighten up through the phone line as they begin to picture another possibility. They typically say, "This is the best conversation I have had since this whole nightmare began."

I then go on to explain that their diagnosis is not a negative thing; it is simply their body's way of expressing a weakness or deficiency in some area. Cancer doesn't come out of the blue, it doesn't just pop up in a random spot of the body without good reason, and it can't simply be removed without looking at the whole picture. It is an encompassing disease that requires the body's defense mechanism to kick in—the physical structure and emotional environment must be addressed and treated, not just the disease.

When cancer cells form in a healthy body, they are recognized by the strong immune system and quickly eliminated before becoming a problem. Tumors typically grow slowly, giving the body time to gather its defenses. This is good news for us; we simply need to restore our health on an emotional, physical, and energetic level. That's not so tough—I know exactly how to do it! Been there and done that. Remember, go with your first instinct and gut intuition, as it's typically the correct one. Know that for every problem, there is a natural solution. And above all, remember: *You can do this.*

When the shit hit the fan for me, I knew I had to begin asserting myself and become proactive. I spent hours, weeks, months, and years on research, discovering new alternative modalities so I could empower myself with tools to get in shape for the fight of my life. Would you compete in the Olympics, climb Mount Everest, or play in the Super Bowl without appropriate training or the proper tools and equipment? No, you would not. The diagnosis you have been given is your challenge. It requires you to be in peak condition. This is your call to action. If your life were a movie, how would you want it to turn out?

Be the hero, stand up, and let everyone (including yourself) know that you're here and present, ready to kick some ass.

Stay Out of the Victim Trap

I always say "the cancer." I never say "my cancer"— I do not claim it as something I own. When others say "your cancer," as if they're tagging you with it, correct them by simply stating, "It's not *my* cancer. It's *the* cancer, and it's leaving my body now." Empower yourself with your words; others will follow your lead. Never take on a victim role or operate from a place of defeat.

When you find out you have cancer, your first instinct may be to tell everyone you know. Be careful, since people can become like rapidly dividing cancer cells and spread your news out of control. As the story gets passed along from person to person, it can become overdramatized and distorted, like the childhood game of telephone. Steer clear of those individuals who like to be saviors (or as I call them, the "brisket brigade"). They'll keep stopping by to commiserate over your tragic situation, almost as if they want to keep you mired down in the muck of your "bad news." Some of the things people said to me left me in utter dismay . . . maybe it made them feel better about their own lives.

There is certainly a place for allowing others to comfort you while you process the overwhelming wave of emotions that accompanies a diagnosis; however, you absolutely must avoid those who keep you in the "Poor, Pitiful Pearl" program. This would not be healthy for you. Even so, it's very easy to fall into the "victim trap"—in which you find that it behooves you to stay sick because it defines who you are.

I quickly discovered that I didn't have time to wallow and feel sorry for myself. There was too much work to be done. I remember the surprise on one of my neighbor's faces when I greeted him one day with a huge smile and upbeat attitude. He went on about the horror of it all, while I reported how great I felt and thanked him for visiting me. He almost seemed defeated when he couldn't save me.

Another time, I received a sympathy/condolence card from someone I barely knew. I remember asking my husband when I opened it, "Who died?" On the flip side, a friend of mine gave me a card that was so powerful and positive, telling me that if there was anyone equipped to deal with this challenge and kick ass, it was me. I loved that card. For anyone reading this who wonders how to console a loved one struggling with cancer, remember that the person doesn't need sympathy—but rather, strength, encouragement, optimism, or maybe simply an ear.

Ask for What You Need and Create Your Own Support Team

I was so used to taking care of others, being fully competent, and managing everyone's lives—so many people had depended on me to "fix it"—that accepting any type of help was extremely difficult for me. When a very dear friend asked if she could bring me groceries, it was such a struggle for me to say yes. I just couldn't allow someone else to do the caretaking. But my friend didn't give up, calmly telling me, "Dena, let someone help you. Let someone take care of you . . . it's okay."

Finally, I was able to say, "Yes, thank you." I started to practice that answer, and to use it more often. I learned that there is nothing wrong with accepting help from friends and family, or asking for it when you need to.

Most people don't know what to do or say, so it will be a learning curve for everyone involved. All you have to do is ask for what you need from a place of appreciation and gratitude, and allow the ones who care about you to be the blessing they are.

You'll need a support team—mine was called "Team D." Some of them helped me with natural cooking so that I could eat a strict diet of macrobiotic food. Others came with me to chemo treatments and talked me through guided meditation and visualization. Still others were there to shower me with thoughtful little gifts and acts of kindness when I needed it most. One friend even helped me create a vision board with positive messages, such as: *I have decided to become fully conscious; I love myself unconditionally;* and *I am healthy, whole, and free to let go of the past.*

11

I am grateful to all the members of my team who rallied and helped me kick cancer's ass. I bless them all.

In the beginning, I also really wanted to be around someone who had gone through what I was about to endure, but I didn't know anybody who had. I prayed to my higher power for guidance, and my prayers were answered when I met Vicki, my partner in wellness.

One day I was at Whole Foods Market when I saw a young, happy bald woman. I said, "Hey, Baldy." She was a little taken aback, until I told her that I'd soon be bald, too. We hit it off; and we went on to meet every week for our "no dairy, no wheat, no gluten," seasonally correct, organic meals while downing shots of wheatgrass.

Even though our personal lives were completely opposite, Vicki was someone I could relate to on the cancer level. On days when I knew I had to leave her to endure another treatment, I would hold on to her for dear life. Together, we grew healthier and stronger—and then, when our treatments were finished, we went our separate ways with love and gratitude in our hearts.

In finding companionship through your ordeal, don't try too hard. When I was diagnosed again, I asked my doctor for "another Vicki"—that is, a patient I could relate to or find comfort in—and the patient he connected me with was dying. Ultimately, I felt more depressed than uplifted. I firmly believe that the people you need appear exactly when you need them, as Vicki did for me. (Note that Imerman Angels is a great resource for people who are looking to make what I call a "cancer connection": **www.imermanangels.org**.)

My children gave me great strength as well. I'll never forget when my then-five-year-old son, Jet, told me, "Mom, I was reading a study today." That in itself made me laugh, but he continued, "It said if you laugh and smile more, you'll live longer." He decided that he was going to tell me a joke every day. So at night, I'd ask him, "What time is it, Jet?" He'd say, "It's time to laugh, Mom." Even if I didn't feel like laughing, we would fake it until we could make it. Every single day, no matter how stupid I felt, I laughed so hard with him that tears streamed down my face.

In addition, my stepson Brice brought me DVDs of his favorite comedians, like Dane Cook . . . he's hysterical. My daughter, Paris, learned how to cook healthy favorites and has been a great friend and companion through it all. My oldest stepson, August, made great music CDs. Everyone pitched in to make my recovery a positive one.

Now that you've learned everything you can about your diagnosis, found a patient and supportive doctor, written it all down, and created your positive support team, it's time for the next step. You're ready to grasp the nuts and bolts of cancer treatments.

CHAPTER TWO

The Nuts and Bolts of Treatments, Protocols, and Procedures

Hearing the word *cancer* will typically come when you least expect it. It will blindside you as it knocks you down for the count. Then, as you regain your footing, you'll find yourself in a world where everyone seems to be speaking a foreign language.

I was in my mid-30s when I had to learn how to navigate the complex and frightening world of cancer protocols and procedures. One decade later, I'm not afraid. I am empowered, and you can be, too. So pull yourself together, gather your wits, and grab your notebook and pen.

Rather than try to tackle every possible type of cancer diagnosis and what protocols each one will entail, I'm only going to talk about the treatments and procedures relating to my own personal experience. With that being said, these procedures and protocols are often applicable to other types of cancer as well. (For further in-depth information on the particular cancer you'd like to address, please take a look at the National Cancer Institute's helpful website, the A to Z List of Cancers: **www.cancer.gov /cancertopics/types/alphalist.** For the alternative explanation, you can read a couple of my favorite books, Michio Kushi's *The Cancer Prevention Diet* and Hulda Regehr Clark's *The Cure For All Cancers,* which shed light on the whys and hows of both disease and prevention for every possible diagnosis.)

Detection, Tests, and Scans

Let's start at the beginning, where most diagnoses start: detection. Now, there is no simple test for cancer— you cannot go in for a quick blood test or culture and get a positive or negative result. There are literally thousands of types of cancer, and it can be like assembling a complicated puzzle. After extensive testing and more testing, as well as consulting with many specialists, you might finally figure it out—and even then, there's the possibility of a misdiagnosis. Yep, cancer is complex. As we try to maneuver between the radiologists, imaging/lab technicians, pathologists, and anesthesiologists, there are so many intricacies involved that we could go crazy.

Personally, I believe scans and x-rays can be done too often. I think the medical establishment puts fear out there, and we buy into it hook, line, and sinker. To that end, on a recent episode of his show, Dr. Mehmet Oz spoke about the possible link between thyroid cancer, which is one of the fastest growing cancers in women, and mammograms and x-rays. Dr. Oz actually suggested that people ask for thyroid guards during mammograms and scans. He also demonstrated how dental aprons, used to protect our children and ourselves against the toxic effects of x-rays, should have a flap that reaches up to protect the thyroid. I go even further now and ask for an apron to protect my lower torso when I get a chest x-ray. We *all* must request adequate protection.

Then there are CAT scans, which send out a thin x-ray beam to a number of different points around the body, thus showing a more thorough cross section of the body than a typical x-ray does. Once when I had one of these done, I actually felt like I was being poisoned. I could feel the radiation everywhere, even in my teeth. I felt nauseated and dizzy, and knew that it was penetrating my whole body. Although the doctors told me that this was impossible, every ounce of my being told me, *No more CAT scans for a while.* I didn't have another scan for two years, and I'm still here to talk about it.

When doctors request scans every week or even monthly, I feel it can lead to too much radiation. I mean, really, what's changing? You know the cancer is there, and you must get rid of it. That's all you need to know. When the cancer grew in my body, I had side effects such as pain radiating down my arm, numbness in my hand, and trouble taking a full breath. As the tumor started to shrink, I knew that, too. I don't need a scan to have a sense of myself. I always know when I have cancer. My intuition is typically right—my doctor is always amazed when I know before he does. So I've refused to take all the scans they request. I pick and choose what works for me. All I have to do is listen.

Try this exercise: Notice everything you feel from the cancer. What part of your body is it affecting? Is it hard to breathe? Does your neck hurt? Or is it your stomach or back? Go right there, where the cancer is, and be with it.

Don't be afraid to gain a sense of what cancer feels like so you know yourself. If it comes back, or when it starts to shrink and go away, you can be the first to know. When the cancer metastasized into my bones and lungs, I certainly felt it. I also knew when it was going, going, gone.

I know you're probably thinking, *I'm scared to refuse the doctors' orders.* And I don't blame you—I was scared, too. Yet I have learned over the past ten years to follow my intuition and inner guides, and you will, too. At this point in my cancer career, it has become more like a dance between my doctor and me: These days, my oncologist knows better than to argue with me for the most part, unless he's trying to make a specific point, and then he calmly tells me his reasoning without fear and drama. I respect and trust that he takes my lifestyle into consideration when we make mutual decisions for my health care. I've retrained my doctor to respect the sense I have of myself to the point where he allows me to make some of my own rules in terms of scans and treatments.

I'm not advocating that you avoid scans altogether. Scans are important for early detection and are a necessary part of cancer; without them, we'd be in big trouble. I'm just suggesting you might *limit* them. When I do have any type of scan, I protect myself by using visualizing techniques such as imagining white light or a violet flame of protection all around and through me.

Needle Biopsy and Lumpectomy

If you have a suspicious lump in your breast, typically you will be given a choice of either a needle biopsy or a lumpectomy. In either case, make sure you request the results from your doctor within three days after the procedure. Also, ask your doctor before either the lumpectomy or biopsy if he will be available to schedule a follow-up surgery the next week, *not longer,* if the results are cancerous. (If your doctor won't accommodate your request, find another one who will.) If the needle biopsy or lumpectomy shows malignancy/cancer—especially if the tumor they have removed looks to be encapsulated, which they very often are—the procedure could have broken the encapsulation and released the cancer cells into your body. I don't care how much they say this cannot happen. I suffer today from this mistake.

For my first diagnosis, the tumor in my breast was so small that I chose a routine lumpectomy. The "pea" would be out, and I would be done and go about my business as if this whole thing never happened. I felt a lumpectomy was really no big deal, but I was still nervous about the outcome. For me, there were few physical or emotional repercussions from my lumpectomy. These days, they are so common . . . even so, it is always scary when you hear those dreaded words from your doctor: "Something suspicious."

Insist upon a frozen-section biopsy of your lumpectomy. I didn't, and this is my greatest regret. What this means is that while you're under anesthesia, the doctors will freeze the mass they've taken out and quickly analyze it before finishing the operation, in order to make sure they've removed the entire tumor and you have clean margins. You'd rather that they take the time right then to ensure they got out all the cancer instead of waiting to discover this weeks later. This is the most important piece of life-saving information you should know about your lumpectomy.

You are the customer, you are paying all of these medical professionals, and you can ask for whatever you need. *Use your voice.* Had I known about conducting a frozen section at the time of my initial lumpectomy, it likely would have saved me from what I was to endure for the rest of my life. How in the hell could that first surgeon have left unclean margins on a one-millimeter tumor? When I asked him about it, he replied, "You didn't request a frozen section." Was that my job? Was I really supposed to know what that was and know to request that from him?

If they don't get clean margins from the lumpectomy, even with the frozen section—which can happen—you will be exposed to roaming cancer cells. After all I've witnessed, my humble opinion is that a mastectomy should be scheduled immediately. *Do not wait!*

In all the years I've been dealing with cancer, I've seen one common denominator: after a possible leak or spread of cells by way of needle biopsy or lumpectomy, chemotherapy and radiation will not be enough. The women who remove their breast have the best chance of remaining cancer free. I wish I'd removed mine right from the beginning, but then again, hindsight is always 20/20.

Surgery

After a lumpectomy or needle biopsy that tests positive for cancer, schedule surgery as soon as possible. It was a total of seven weeks from the time of my lumpectomy until I could clean up the remaining cancer cells in my breast. My intuition told me this was too long to wait, and the disease could be spreading everywhere. I was very upset, but I felt I had no choice. *Never* wait that long to remove cancer that's been released into your body.

I've watched plenty of surgeries and been the recipient of more. I know firsthand how debilitating it can be, as I always spend the first few hours throwing up from anesthesia. It was also disturbing to know that through most of my surgeries, I was strapped to a board for hours. No wonder I felt as if I'd been beaten up like a piece of luggage afterward.

I now give doctors my laundry list of requests, letting them know that I'm an old pro at the surgery game. I bring my healing music so they can play it during surgery. I tell them to keep me warm—after all, I'm sleeping, not dead. I sweetly ask them to be gentle with me, as I am as sensitive as a butterfly. They laugh when I tell them that I will feel it after surgery if they abuse me, and I will hunt them down and make them pay for it. When giving me anesthesia, I insist that less is truly more with me. I also let them know that my subconscious can hear everything, so I ask that they only say positive things. They are usually very accommodating.

Although it can be difficult, you must ask for what you need. Even when you do assert yourself, it can fall on deaf ears, as the medical establishment seems to think they know you better than you know yourself. Stay tough.

A Cautionary Tale

After one of my surgeries, I couldn't get a breath in. I told them something was wrong, but they brushed me off. Then they discovered that my lung had been punctured during surgery. To fix it, I had to undergo a hellacious experience as a tube was inserted into my chest, through my rib cage, and into my lung—while awake. As you might know, you can't eat for a 12-hour period before surgery due to the risk of vomiting . . . and I'd already eaten ice chips and applesauce right after I was initially operated on. So they now refused to give me any anesthesia for the lung procedure, which involved strapping me down and cutting a hole in my chest. What kept going through my mind was how awful it must have been for Holocaust victims. The torture they endured made me feel like I could somehow get through this.

After I'd been up all night with a tube sticking into my lung, I still couldn't breathe. I tried to tell the surgeon, but he said, "You're fine," and yanked the tube from my chest. I gasped for air. Sure enough, two hours later, I couldn't breathe again. A gentler doctor did the procedure once again. What a difference a caring physician can make.

Healing After Surgery

After all surgeries, you need to put the pieces back together again, like Humpty Dumpty. Use all the help you can find, such as lymph-drainage practitioners, massage therapists, acupuncturists, foot reflexologists, and craniosacral therapists (see Chapter 3 for more details). Also, try exercises you can do on your own, such as tai chi, yoga, dance, and swimming. Do anything you can to get the blood flowing and the lymphatic system circulating. And drink plenty of water and healing teas to help cleanse the body from post-surgery toxins.

Depletion along with depression are common side effects after surgery. I can relate it to a movie or video game where one person is getting annihilated or beaten to a pulp, but as soon as he pulls himself up with that "killer look" in his eyes, the crowd goes wild. Doesn't it feel great when you're watching this kind of movie or playing this type of game, watching the hero get up on his feet, ready for battle? This can be you! Imagine that you are that warrior, beating the living hell out of the enemy. If you aren't in great shape, there's no time like now to get your ass in gear and be that hero.

People ask me how I escaped depression—after all, I'd been through hell and back. I tell them that all the natural remedies and treatments I incorporate in my life, not to mention "clean food" (more about this type of food in Chapter 5), helped tremendously. They really work. You see, besides its psychological affects, surgery depletes the energy of the kidneys/bladder, liver, spleen, gallbladder, and lungs. Whenever I have surgery, I tend to awaken with congestion in my lungs. So I take pleurisy root to support the lungs, and I use the incentive spirometer given to me by the hospital. I don't take the ugly little blue socks home with me, but I do take that "little breathing buddy," which helps strengthen the lungs.

I suggest you gather your team and all the tools you will need *before* surgery. I ask friends to bring miso soup and healing foods so I don't have to eat poor-quality hospital food. I also ask my natural practitioners to come visit me. I once found an acupuncturist offered through the hospital. No one's going to tell you if you don't ask—so ask, ask, ask.

Sentinel-Node Biopsy/Lymph-Node Dissection

The sentinel node is known as the "protector," and is the first lymph node that filters the fluid that drains away from the breast. Thus, if a surgeon can remove the sentinel node and it is cancer free, then it is very likely that the other nodes are not affected. In the past, doctors removed ten or more lymph nodes to excavate any possible cancerous nodes; now, researchers use "technetium 99 scintigraphy" or "blue dye" injection to assess the extent of node involvement. I wish this had been available for me, but it wasn't; instead, the surgeon removed 22 nodes to find that 2 were affected. Having my lymph nodes removed was not only the most painful of surgeries, but it was also the most heartbreaking. I was not prepared for the news when I awoke: I had to face chemotherapy.

Before I talk about that, though, I want to tell you about one of the horrific side effects of lymph-node dissections: a condition called lymphedema, which is localized fluid retention due to insufficient lymphatic drainage. For women dealing with breast cancer, this means swollen arms or chest; for other kinds of cancer, there may be swelling in other areas.

The lymphatic system is a network of tissues, organs, and vessels that help maintain the body's fluid balance. Our immune system, along with all of our organs, is connected to a network of lymphatic vessels that parallel the functions of the body's veins and arteries. Due to the intricacies of this "web," the lymphatic system plays a key role in our health and overall immune function.

To keep your lymphatic system running efficiently, you need to stretch the arm that has been operated on. Don't let the energy in your arm stay constricted—open up the entire area and expand your wings so you can fly, little birdie, fly. This is not a matter to be taken lightly. So many women end up with a big, swollen arm or what's known as "frozen shoulder." You must kick your own ass here. There is a fine line between overprotecting and knowing how much you can really push yourself.

The day after they removed the surgical drain in my breast, I started stretching my adjacent arm with specific shoulder-opening exercises on doorjambs and on the floor (videos of these exercises are available on my website). As soon as I felt ready, I began practicing yoga, and I learned all the ways that I could gently but assertively release scar tissue and gain full motion back in my wounded arm. I also saw a lymph-drainage master who helped stimulate my lymphatic system with special exercises.

Other methods to prevent lymphedema and promote lymph drainage include dancing, swimming, and jumping on the trampoline. Cardio exercises before and after surgery help keep the lymphatic system moving. If you don't work on opening your arm and stretching it out, you could restrict your range of motion. Stagnant scar tissue may lead to back, neck, and shoulder problems.

Chemotherapy

When my husband went through chemo for bile-duct cancer, I remember so clearly saying to him, "I'm just glad it's you and not me because I couldn't do it." The needles and drugs that made him so sick and depleted scared the hell out of me. So when it was my turn, I came up with my own plan to prepare for it.

I knew that I'd eventually be bald, so I cut off my long hair. I also wanted to do something fun and childlike before I had to face the torment of this treatment. What's the opposite of a torture chamber? Disney World. That's right—my husband and I ditched school with the kids and ran away, without a care, to Florida. We went on every ride and sang every song.

When we returned to Chicago, I started the nightmare of my life. Initially, I was prescribed a chemotherapy protocol called Adriamycin Cytoxan (AC). According to my doctors, it was the "standard of care" for breast cancer. As there weren't any other options, they prescribed a "one size fits all" treatment and hoped it would have some effect.

My healthy body did not like chemotherapy one bit. I was violently ill after the first treatment. I couldn't eat or drink, so I had to have a nurse come to my home to administer IV fluids. Being knocked down by a chemo that was so invasive, destructive, and depleting—but had virtually no effect on the cancer they were trying to treat—didn't give me much of a chance. The wrong chemo was the last thing my already-compromised immune system needed.

"This isn't the right chemo for me," I told my husband. "I know it isn't working . . . what it's doing is killing me." I didn't grow the guts I needed to say no until later, after years of following along like a helpless lemming.

After almost a year, which seemed like forever, I got through four treatments with the help of my very dear friend Vicki (whom I mentioned in Chapter 1), who was 30 years old and going through the same thing as I was at the same time.

I also found a natural doctor who revived me after each treatment. He came to my house and worked on my depleted liver, digestive system, and ravaged kidneys. He worked his magic by using Shiatsu and other Asian-based modalities to unblock energy pathways. God bless him for being there for me. One of the things I noticed through my health-awakening experience is: "When the student is ready, the teacher appears." This has been so true for me throughout this entire amazing and incredible health-awakening journey. . . .

After chemo, I explored breath work, did a lot of yoga, and ate clean/healing foods. Chemotherapy not only stressed my liver, as it had to filter the toxins, but it also left me feeling frustrated and angry. I was no stranger to these emotions, but after chemo, they seemed magnified. I started to see a clear connection between tightness in my liver and deep, unresolved resentment and anger issues— and I realized that my liver needed a break, physically and emotionally.

During this time, I found Louise Hay's baby blue "bible," *Heal Your Body*. It cleverly explained the emotional connection between symptoms and illness, and assisted me in much of my emotional work. I wrote Louise's affirmations for cancer on every mirror in the house, for example: *I love and approve of myself,* and *I freely forgive and let go of the past.* (I recommend this little lifesaving book to all my clients, no matter the malady.)

To chemo or not to chemo? It's really a case-by-case decision. My chemo was not right for me; my husband's chemo saved his life. I'm lucky to have lived long enough to see the invention of targeted drug therapies like Herceptin, the one I am on today. Yet if chemotherapy is the correct regimen for you, it can be a very good thing. Just do your research and trust your intuition.

PICC Line/Subcutaneous Port

I wish someone had told me to get a PICC line or a subcutaneous port before I started chemotherapy. These are devices that doctors implant under your skin in your arm or chest so they can gain direct access to your veins without destroying them. A PICC (peripherally inserted central catheter) is inserted into the arm; a port can be placed in the chest or arm, and it doesn't dangle outside the body the way a PICC does. Either can be implanted for a long period of time—nurses can use them to draw blood samples and to administer liquids such as chemotherapy and IV fluids without needing to stick a needle in a new vein each time.

When I was making my rounds like a zombie to different doctors, listening to the various options regarding my treatment protocol, I certainly wasn't interested in any added surgeries or in having a foreign object inserted in my already-traumatized body. I chose not to use a PICC line or a port, and I couldn't have been more wrong. By the end of my fourth treatment, my veins were so damaged from stringent chemotherapy drugs that I could never access them again.

During subsequent diagnoses, I chose to insert a port into my chest. What an amazing gift. I can't stress enough how this port has saved my life in terms of the monthly Herceptin treatments I receive, any testing in which I have to be injected with dyes, and my weekly vitamin infusions (further description in Chapter 4).

I happen to be very thin, so my port is easy to see as it protrudes out of my chest and sort of looks like an On/Off button for some kind of futuristic robot. When my children catch other kids staring at my port, they respond in a matter-of-fact tone, "When our mom talks too much, we simply press her Off button for a while." Then they press my "button" and I go quiet, playing along with their little game.

If you are just about to begin chemotherapy of any kind and are questioning whether to get a port or not, I suggest you get one. I personally think it would be so much easier if we were all born with them; it would save countless nervous trips to the doctor for routine blood work or any kind of shot.

Radiation

Radiation therapy relies on targeted radiation beams to kill cancer cells. Just like chemotherapy, radiation targets fast-growing cancer cells. I went for one treatment, but I couldn't bear to go back. It was too traumatizing. Although they called it "low dose," I felt it in my teeth, my ears, and my heart. It even started to constrict my esophagus. I knew instinctively that it would have a negative long-term effect on me. The doctors said this was impossible, but I (as usual) was sensitive, and I knew what I felt.

Although my intuition was screaming at me, I still wasn't sure whether to go back for the ten additional treatments. I really struggled with this dilemma. I went inside my heart during a meditation session to look for the answer, and sure enough, it came that night. I dreamed I was yelling at all my clients, who were lined up like lemmings ready to go through this Dr. Seuss–like machine to get radiated. I was screaming, "Don't do it!" They couldn't hear me, so I yelled louder, "*Do not* follow them in there! It isn't right for you! Don't believe them!" I awoke and knew the answer. I never went back for another treatment.

As I write this book, it's been exactly two years since then, and I just had my fourth brain scan. Although I feel I made the correct decision for myself about radiation, every situation is completely different, and you'll have to choose what is right for *you*. For those of you who opt for radiation, there are plenty of protocols that will protect and help heal any side effects you may encounter.

Radiation can be far-reaching in terms of how it affects other areas of the body. Many of my clients come to me with burning of the esophageal and stomach linings from radiation of the breast, throat, or abdomen. I combine liquid aloe vera and Glutagenics—a product made by Metagenics that has glutamine, licorice-root extract, and aloe-leaf extract—for them, which I mix with water and have them drink two to three times a day. (See "Remedies for Radiation Therapy" in Appendix B.) In fact, whenever my digestion is compromised or I experience burning of the esophageal and stomach lining, I drink this soothing aloe cocktail—and poof! It works. The best part is that it doesn't cause 15 other side effects like prescribed medications do.

When going through radiation, it's imperative to mix arnica gel, Traumeel gel, and Bach Rescue Remedy together as a topical cream for the area being burned by radiation. (You can also use them as an internal treatment; again, see Appendix B for more information.)

When our bodies are in perfect balance, they reflect the exact same mineral content as the sea. Therefore, I eat lots of seaweed. I find it interesting that, as Hiroko Furo, Ph.D., claims in his article "Dietary Practice of Hiroshima/ Nagasaki Atomic Bomb Survivors," a diet based in the traditional Japanese and miso-enriched foods helped survivors of the Nagasaki and Hiroshima atomic bombs and minimized the side effects of radiation.

I realize your doctor might not offer this information. Or he may have told you that natural remedies could hinder your chances to cure cancer. I can only say what I know from my experiences, and that's why I recommend these radiation remedies. I successfully used the gel concoction on my husband's stomach when he was undergoing radiation, and it prevented burning and helped with his recovery.

Mastectomy and Reconstructive Surgery

In the musical I wrote, *Standard of Care,* I described what it was like to have a mastectomy. I wrote it from the perspective of my right breast: "I try to imagine what it might be like to hug a chest without us. When you hug your best friend or your sister, we are the first things you feel; we are the warmth behind every hug. When a child skins their knee or feels scared, they run to their mother's bosom, where they find comfort and safety. In a woman's bosom, you find all her strength and all her soft, feminine beauty. We are heroes."

I chose to have a straightforward mastectomy. The night before surgery, I blessed my perfect, beautiful breast for all the giving it had done and for feeding both my healthy children. I thanked it for all its hard work in mothering, caretaking, and nurturing. I've come to love my new breast. My body is perfect with it.

I have seen various results from breast reconstructions, and have found that the most beautiful results come from straightforward reconstructions without disturbing the abdomen or shoulder. In these instances, a flap of tissue is used from either the belly or back to create a breast mound. In the end, you will have to decide what is best for you and your body, but to make more of a mess in terms of surgical wounds was not my idea of fun—less is sometimes more. I ultimately tattooed a butterfly where an areola would be. This signified my metamorphosis and growth. This loss in my life turned out to be the death of the old and a beautiful rebirth, like a butterfly.

Women who coddle their new breasts, shoulder, and arm like an overprotective parent will not see the best results from their mastectomy. Stagnation may also lead to frozen shoulder. I found that by massaging my mastectomy breast, it eventually started to move more like my real one. And by opening my shoulder, chest, and back with exercises, I could release the scar tissue in the breast area. Don't be afraid to get to know your new breast. Touch, massage, and really feel it; be creative in tattooing it, if you like. Love both of your beautiful, sexy breasts. Don't hide them.

After removing a breast, doctors typically put expanders in so you don't stretch the skin all at once. It was an amazing transformation to watch my new mastectomy breast get pumped up every week with saline. My kids even came—I involved them as much as I could in the process so it wouldn't be a scary mystery for them.

I certainly don't mean to minimize the experience of losing your breasts, but I can honestly say it was not that traumatic for me. It wasn't a painful process, and I liked my new breast, so I was never overcome with grief. Maybe the overwhelming emotional trauma that came with being diagnosed, the possibility of dying, and then going through the toxic hell of chemo, overshadowed any major physical or emotional side effects from losing my breast.

Metastases

When cancer spreads, it's known as a "metastasis." The tumor may spread via lymph or blood to another area of the body.

I was having trouble breathing and thought I had a spasm in my back. I went to the chiropractor every week for an adjustment—it turns out that my alignment wasn't the issue. The cancer had spread from the tiny node in my breast to my neck, bones, and lungs. Thank goodness the first metastasis was four years after the initial lumpectomy. My doctor said he couldn't believe it took that long to show up again, and that I must be doing something right. The type of cancer I had was very aggressive, but due to my healthy lifestyle, I kept it at bay.

I started on the Herceptin, along with another type of chemotherapy called Vinorelbine. I responded so well that it only took about four weeks to rid my body of cancer. Targeted drug therapies are amazing, but unfortunately they've only been created for certain types of cancer. The premise behind them is that they only attack cancer cells so as to not completely destroy the whole body or healthy cells in the process. Although these drugs were easier to tolerate, and the doctors said they were totally benign, I still felt some repercussions. I've come to learn that no medicine is totally benign, and you're foolish if you believe it is.

Four years after the bone, lung, and neck diagnosis, I experienced the loss of feeling in my left pinky. As always, I was in tune to my body's signs. I was under a tremendous amount of stress in my life, so the doctors wrote my symptoms off to that, but I knew better.

One night I had one of my intuitive dreams telling me there was trouble ahead. And then my dog, whom I'd saved from a shelter ten years earlier, started sleeping next to my side of the bed after always sleeping in the kitchen. I woke up one morning and stepped on him. I asked him, "Woody, am I dying, boy? Why are you sleeping right next to me?" He didn't answer, but I saw it in his eyes. He sensed danger was coming, as dogs typically do.

When I had a seizure, it was so painful that I actually thought I was having a stroke. I prayed for God's white light. God answered me right before I lost consciousness with a vision of my brother, Bradley, who had died five years earlier. He was so beautiful, with a golden luminescence. I asked him if I was going to see my kids again, and Bradley said, "Yes, Dena. It is not your time; you have more work to do. You have a brain tumor. It is not meant to hurt you; it will be easy to remove."

Finding out that I had a brain tumor hit me like a ton of bricks. Yet although it was an eight-hour surgery, it was easy to remove as far as brain tumors go.

I felt instinctively that the Herceptin had stopped working for me. I was right. A week after the brain surgery, I felt a small nodule in my neck and demanded a PET scan. It turns out that the cancer had metastasized to another area—like a bad sequel, the lump was back. Had I built up immunity to the drug that had once worked so well?

I continued on the Herceptin and started more chemo, the same chemo they had put me on for lung and bone cancer four years earlier. I did four rounds when we realized it wasn't doing anything but depleting me. I was seriously becoming resistant to all this shit, and I knew it.

What I needed was to stop depending on drugs that had a shelf life and to go back to what I was sure would work, back to building my immune system the old-fashioned way. I was determined to find a new protocol by searching out more diverse modalities, remedies, and healers . . . which takes us on a whirlwind journey across the country in the next chapter.

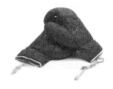

CHAPTER THREE

The Great and Powerful Oz: Elixirs, Gurus, Guides, and Modalities

Just making decisions about your overall health-care plan can be stressful. And, as I detailed in the last chapter, it can be challenging to navigate through treatments, protocols, and procedures when you're diagnosed with cancer. However, there are plenty of ways to make all of this easier on you both physically and emotionally, using complementary medicine. In fact, I've seen people with certain types of cancer go into remission by changing their diet and using a variety of alternative modalities to decrease inflammation and boost their immune system.

Once again, you'll have to find things that resonate with you, and follow your own intuition. I personally learned to treat healing practices in the same way I've always treated religion: I take a little from here, a little from there, and mix it all up to create what works for me. I find beauty in all religions, as I do in the wide array of therapeutic modalities that are available. I promise the answers will come. As you open yourself up to be a receiver, so shall you receive exactly what you need when you need it.

Elixirs

Researchers agree that a healthy diet, along with nutritional supplements, can improve survival chances and stress levels throughout treatment. As Patrick Quillin, author of *Beating Cancer with Nutrition,* writes: "Over 40% of cancer patients actually die from malnutrition, not from the cancer. . . . You cannot fight a life-threatening disease while malnourished. You need all the proper nutrition you can get to feed your immune system, which is your army assigned to killing the cancer cells."

In an ideal world we would get all or most of the vitamins, minerals, and nutrients we need out of our food. However, in today's industrialized world, this is usually not possible, so we must make up for what our food lacks by using supplements. With that being said, I'm not a believer in taxing the body with too many pills that you have to swallow and digest . . . it only burdens your digestive system.

Throughout my journey, remedies have come and gone, depending on how I've felt and what internal organ has needed strengthening or detoxing. Like me, you need to be creative, and don't stay stuck on the same regimen year after year. You may become immune, and your body might even reject some remedies after prolonged use.

When considering what supplements to take, first check in with yourself by asking simple questions: "What do I feel today—am I depleted in something, am I dehydrated, is my digestion stressed, or am I experiencing any pain in my body?" Your protocol will change as you regress during some periods and make progress during others. To that end, I followed my intuition when my natural doctor offered me a shake to clear my liver and rid my body of excess mucus and damp heat created by chemotherapy. I knew it was working, as I could feel and see the mucus leaving my body through every orifice . . . not so attractive. When I no longer needed this shake, I knew that, too.

Out of necessity, I developed what I call my "Cancer Tool Kit." For example, I found that I couldn't live without Chzyme, an herbal supplement made by Health Concerns that acts as a digestive enzyme and helps tremendously with nausea; Ultra Flora Plus DF, which is made by Metagenics and helps build good bacteria in the intestinal tract; and Glutagenics, which, as I mentioned in the last chapter, soothes the esophageal and stomach lining. Due to a suppressed and compromised digestion, I like liquids and powders. (I talk about all these remedies and much more in detail in Appendix B.)

A vitamin infusion is my favorite quick fix. (Remember that port I talked about previously? This is where it comes in handy, as the infusions are administered intravenously.) I suggested this treatment to a client looking to rebuild her ravaged immune system. When she asked her doctor for a prescription, since insurance companies may cover part of the cost, he said, "We offer them here at the hospital." She looked at him in utter disbelief—and then, with all the anger this 4'11", 90-pound, 80-year-old woman could muster, shouted, "Are telling me that you have been torturing me with this chemo for four years, and now you tell me you can give me some vitamins?!"

Again, it's amazing what doesn't automatically occur to doctors. I've often had medical professionals ask me what I ate or did to stay in such great shape. They've been impressed by the fact that my heart stayed strong, I had healthy white- and red-blood-cell counts, I didn't lose my menstrual cycle as predicted, and I never looked sick. I also bounced back quickly after all my surgeries. Much of this is thanks to my commitment to nutrition and my devout willingness to not only learn about, but to try, any and all herbs, tinctures, and protocols; along with my quest to uncover the world's supreme healers, gurus, and guides. (They should really make a reality-TV show out of this.)

Gurus and Guides

> **Guru:** one who is regarded as having great knowledge, skill, wisdom, and authority in a certain area and who uses it to guide others (teacher); in Sanskrit, *gu* means "darkness" and *ru* means "light"; a spiritual master leads you out of the darkness and into the light.
>
> **Guide:** one who shows the way by leading, directing, or advising; he or she serves as a model for others.

I think of gurus as people who devote their lives to bestowing their vast wisdom and knowledge upon others as a lifelong sharing journey. These natural-born healers and generous spirits are not looking for monetary fulfillment or notoriety; they're simply following their destiny to lead other men and women out of the pain of the human experience. Guides, on the other hand, are individuals whom you engage or pay to advise, teach, or direct you by offering different physical modalities and/or supplement protocols. Both groups use their intuitive healing energies and education to help the best way they can.

I've had many gurus and guides over the past decade— some living, and some who have long since passed and left only their words. One of the first was Paramahansa Yogananda, author of *Autobiography of a Yogi*, who taught me how powerful our minds can be and how we possess self-healing gifts. When Yogananda wrote about the guides he was privileged to study under, it made me that much hungrier to seek out a guru. Through Yogananda's understanding of his own guru's death, I learned that dying can be a beautiful thing and should not be feared. This idea was liberating to me because I'd just lost my dear, sweet brother, and I always feared death myself. I recommend this book to anyone facing an exit from this Earth plane (a death).

Some of the gurus and guides I've worked with have had a huge influence on my ability to not only heal myself, but others. I found amazing teachers who generously shared their magical bodywork and remedy protocols with me, teaching me about the "art of living" and the power of breath work. My nurturing colon hydrotherapist gently detoxified me, and I had the privilege of working with an intuitive lymph-drainage master and a talented kinesiologist from Belgium.

Some healers you meet on your journey might simply be guides who help you with a specific problem, while others seem to be sent from above; it's divine inspiration. You know when you've met one, and you cannot possibly try to make it happen—it sort of falls into place. It's synchronistic the way planets align themselves to fit your needs. I believe this happens when your angels or higher spirit guides work together to send you a gift.

My gift was Max Vanorman, who is a natural healer and my own personal guru. He has had the most influence on my life, beginning when I first went to him at the ripe old age of 17 for help with my chronic stomach issues. From the years I spent on Max's table, I received many pearls of wisdom. And whenever I read a great book or hear a brilliant speaker on the subject of cancer, it never fails—the dietary protocols all look similar to Max's. (I include much of what I learned from him in Chapter 5, which is dedicated to our almighty food.)

I know firsthand that Max's methods work. His first line of defense focuses on healing foods, which means cutting out sugar and overprocessed and chemically laden foods. I will admit that this is *not* easy. That's because we're all addicts: addicts of food, addicts of the "the quick fix," and addicts of momentary pleasure. Some people will say, "It's too hard to give up my sugar, gluten, alcohol, or dairy," even as they're fighting for their lives. You'd think the way they go on and on about their favorite food that they'll actually die without it . . . on the contrary, they'll die *with* it.

It would be impossible to include everything I learned from Max in one book. As I asked him on many occasions, "How can I possibly remember the sheer amount of information you're filling me with?" With his calming smile and ocean-blue eyes, he'd simply say, "You will remember it when you need it." I felt as if I were working with the teacher from the old television series *Kung Fu*.

Following is an abbreviated list of Max's healing instructions:

- Get digestive help in the form of probiotics (acidophilus) to build up good bacteria in the intestines.

- Use essential oregano oil, one of the most powerful antibacterial remedies there is.

- Drink lots of clean, reverse-osmosis water and herb teas, such as cherry bark, licorice, and pleurisy root; and immune-system builders such as echinacea, ginger, and raspberry.

- Eat plenty of warm, nourishing veggie soups and stews.

- Make sure your bowels are emptied daily.

- Avoid all sugars, caffeine, chemicals, and drugs of any kind.

- Avoid soy foods, except fermented soy products such as miso and aged shoyu.

- Keep your feet and extremities warm.

- Reduce the use of pain medication and other prescription drugs as much as possible.

- Reduce stress as much as possible, including overexercising and overthinking.

- Go to bed by 10 P.M.

One day I was overwhelmed by a dilemma in my life, and I sat down to listen to one of Dr. Wayne Dyer's meditation CDs. In the middle of my "ohms," I heard Max's voice, as if he were in the room with me. He said, "Do not debate." This was something he said quite often throughout the years I worked with him, and now I finally understood what he meant.

"Do not debate" means to accept the change that is coming or happening, that our first instinct or intuition is typically the correct one. I had to smile because Max was right as usual. I could never begin to thank him with mere words of gratitude.

You will inevitably come across all types of teachers, gurus, and guides. Some you may not resonate with, while others will move and inspire you. Remember, a mentor can be found anywhere, so be open to the exciting new world that will unfold as you learn to tune in and receive.

Natural Doctors

When I get a diagnosis of cancer, I know what I'm looking for in a physician, and I find the rest in natural doctors. It is, once again, a balance.

What are "natural doctors"? I use the term to describe alternative practitioners who train in specific modalities or genres of healing such as lymph drainage, kinesiology, or acupuncture. They might be naturopathic doctors or those who simply label themselves as holistic health-care providers. It's not about the name; it's about what they offer, how they make you feel, and if they help you heal.

In Chapter 1, I offer tips for choosing a regular doctor as part of your team. In terms of finding natural doctors as guides, the rules of the game are pretty much the same. So here are some tips on finding specific or natural healers with whom you can connect:

- They should be open, warm, and comforting.
- They should explain concepts clearly.
- They should know their craft.
- They should be humble enough to understand the need for other health-care providers as a part of your overall health plan.

Since more people today are combining alternative therapies with traditional medicine, you're bound to receive reliable recommendations from friends and family. If you haven't honed your own intuition quite yet, though, I suggest beginning your alternative health-care journey with a great kinesiologist. He or she will be able to help you determine what your specific needs are based on muscle testing.

I know it can be frustrating if your traditional doctor refuses to explore alternative remedies that really work. In a perfect world, regular doctors would be expected to learn more about complementary/alternative modalities. If regular doctors and alternative healers came together to make love, not war, our lives would take a dramatic turn for the best. Physicians would soon realize that it is more important to know what type of person has the disease than what type of disease the person has. Bottom line, we are not defined by our disease. We don't need to focus on the problem or deficit, but we need to understand how to nourish the natural abundance of our health.

One day while shopping for antiques, I came across a book written in the 19th century called *The Regulars*. The book distinguished between two types of healers. On the one hand, there were the Regulars, who developed what they call "sophisticated science," which included medicines that not only killed disease, but also suppressed the entire immune system. The Naturals, on the other hand, were healers who used many of the same remedies and modalities that I use for my family today—such as oregano oil as an antibacterial, olive oil and garlic for ear infections, marshmallow root to soothe the stomach, and cherry bark for upper respiratory infections. The Regulars labeled the Naturals as quacks and witch doctors.

While I read this old book, I laughed in amazement as I realized that not much has changed today. Some physicians unfortunately prevent their patients from exploring alternative therapies or more supportive whole foods due to their lack of knowledge. This is tragic.

Whenever I've asked regular doctors why they don't recommend some of these tried-and-true natural remedies or healthier foods to their patients when they see that they work for me, they've all given me the same answer: there haven't been any studies proving that they work. How sad that some doctors live their lives in test tubes!

While some medical professionals are completely in the dark, offering no help when it comes to alternative therapies, I can't give them all a bad rap. I am truly blessed with my oncologist, who sees the proof in the pudding (that's natural tofu pudding) with me. He is open to allowing alternative modalities to have a place in my combined health-care process.

Check with your doctor—he might know if your hospital is associated with an alternative health-care initiative or if they can refer you to complementary practitioners. You can also look up websites that might lead you to natural doctors in your area; some professional associations have ratings on their list of practitioners or can point you to a specific region in which to search for someone. Try a few different practitioners. You might kiss a few frogs along the way (and don't feel like you need to buy something a natural practitioner recommends every time you see that person). Be patient, though—it is worth it when you find a great one.

Be Your Own Guru

As you look for the ideal natural doctor, remember this famous yogic saying: "Be your own guru." The first step to harnessing the power of the guru within is to sit quietly every day for a little while (through meditation). You will receive the gift of deep *samadhi,* or "one pointedness." It's during these blissful moments that you'll be able to look deep into yourself for answers.

You want to develop your healing prowess so that you may be empowered. Don't just look for someone to fix it for you; instead, follow your inner guide. When gifted healers work on me, for instance, I don't just sit and observe what they're doing—I become an active participant in the healing process, always questioning and hungry to learn how and why my body responds to each method.

Although it's quite a treat to have great healing hands touch me, I eventually learned how to become more self-sufficient so that I could heal myself. Today I connect to my source and use my own energy to heal. I gather energy like a ball in my hands and then direct it toward a place in my body in need of attention. We all have the power to heal ourselves, we need only tap into it.

I like to listen to some of my favorite soothing voices, such as Dr. Wayne Dyer and Pema Chödrön. I also use a "heaven and Earth" healing visualization, which I compiled from a variety of my favorite teachers, to ground and connect me as I tune into my inner voice.

Try it yourself:

Sit on a cushion with a straight spine, and close your eyes. Picture the top of your head opening, like the sunroof of a car. Visualize a flood of bright, warming sunlight coming through the crown of your head, infiltrating and filling every cell of your body. Then picture roots growing from your perineum (the space between your genitals and anus) straight down into the earth, branching out and reaching deep through the grass and soil. Into the gravel, down even deeper, your roots grow until they reach the molten lava at the very core of the earth.

I cannot say it enough: Follow your intuition, dreams, and signs. They are gifts. Speaking of which, one of my favorite books, Paulo Coelho's *The Alchemist,* is about noticing the signs on your path. I have a girlfriend who takes this so seriously that she actually thinks that every sign she sees on every corner or billboard is meant just for her. I told her to stop hogging all the signs and leave some for the rest of us.

One night I dreamed that an ugly chicken foot started growing through my bedroom window. It grew and grew until it was huge. Then spiders started pouring out all over my bedroom and all over me. My dreams are intuitive and show me what I need to see—in this case, I was being told that the cancer had metastasized.

Although my dream was very telling, something was amiss. I felt the profound need to search for a new guru who could shed some light on my emotional conundrum.

One name kept coming up over and over: John of God. So after I finished another round of chemotherapy for lung and bone cancer, I was off to see the wizard in Brazil.

I flew halfway around the world to ask the healer of all healers for guidance. He blessed me with powerful answers. Yet one burning question remained, "Do I still have any cancer?" He didn't say a word; his silence spoke volumes. It was as if he was teaching me about my intuitive power as he let me find the answer in my dream that night. In it, I was hiking up a huge red mountain. At the very top, I saw a scary snake. It was so threatening that I didn't think I would be able to finish my hike. I overcame my fear by killing the snake and climbing to the top. I conquered!

When I woke up in the morning, I knew I had a bit more to go. Most important, I knew what John of God was trying to tell me: I needed to look inward for my answers. I returned home and went for a CAT scan. Sure enough, my dream was right—I had more to go.

Don't forget to follow your intuition and look to yourself as your most powerful guide.

Healing Modalities

I realize that you're dealing with many unfamiliar concepts and treatments right now. You might also be at a place where you can't eat or don't feel like doing much— I was there, too. I started with a bite of brown rice and a few sips of homemade miso broth. I filled my lungs with healing breath, practiced gentle yoga, and found a fab reflexologist.

It's okay to take baby steps until you feel comfortable with your new, healthier lifestyle choices. But I also suggest that you become creative and have fun when exploring the infinite possibilities of new healing modalities. Sitting around feeling sorry for yourself while consuming cookies and downing Diet Coke will only cause more toxic overload and stagnation in terms of your lymphatic system, your digestion, your brain, and all of your organs, as well as fueling the cancer.

Whatever you do, don't beat yourself up if you can't change all at once. Instead of remaining stuck in old, unhealthy ways, embrace fresh ideas so that you can live, thrive, and kick ass. Get up and move, find a new treatment to explore, or try an exotic green vegetable. Gain a new perspective by going to your local botanical gardens as you take a deep breath of fresh air filled with pure gratitude.

Know that there are many modalities to support you on your journey. You can try one or all of them until you find what works for you. Some of the following might be covered by insurance, and some may be free at cancer wellness centers. I love to be a health detective, so I've tried a vast array of them myself:

— **Ayurveda** is grounded in a metaphysics of the "five great elements": *prithvi* (earth), *aap* (water), *tej* (fire), *vaayu* (air), and *akash* (ether). These are the elements that make up the Universe, including the human body. Ayurveda deals with and measures the health during one's entire life span by stressing a balance of three elemental energies or humors: *vata* (wind), *pitta* (bile), and *kapha* (phlegm). According to ayurveda, these three regulatory principles, or doshas, must exist harmoniously for optimal health. Ayurveda says that each human possesses a unique combination of doshas, and when they are in a balanced state, the body will function at its optimal potential.

— **Bioacoustics,** or "life sounds," uses voice spectral analysis and low-frequency sound to eliminate old thought patterns and reintroduce new brain-wave patterns in an effort to help the body rid itself of, or reverse, the disease process.

— **Colon irrigation** (also called "colon hydrotherapy" or "colonics") involves flushing the colon with warm, filtered water. A colonic removes a buildup of waste, which is harmful for digestive and general health. Regular colonics help remove fecal matter that builds up in the colon and interferes with the body's ability to absorb nutrients. (*Please note:* Some individuals should see a doctor before getting a colonic, including people who are pregnant or suffering with Crohn's disease or severe hemorrhoids. I talk more about colonics in Chapter 4.)

— **Craniosacral therapy** works with the spine, skull, diaphragm, and fasciae, releasing restrictions of nerve passages. Craniosacral therapists treat mental stress, neck and back pain, migraines, and temporomandibular joint (or "TMJ") pain; they've also been known to alleviate the chronic pain of fibromyalgia. I received this therapy after my brain surgery, and it was very helpful.

— **Energy psychology** looks at the force that creates problems due to energetic disruptions, which can cause stagnant emotions. There are chemical, neurological, physical, hormonal, and even environmental aspects to emotions. Therefore, the energy psychologist works with the body's bioenergetic systems, including the nervous system, acupuncture meridians, aura, and meridians.

— **Image streaming** is a powerful technique that enables you to find answers by increasing your self-awareness. This technique enables you to attain higher-level thinking and can help you gain a new sense of yourself. Image streaming allows you to look deep into your subconscious mind for answers.

— **Infrared saunas** take detoxification to a whole new level—you can actually sweat toxins out through the skin. Evidence has shown that an infrared sauna can also aid in lowering blood pressure and may help increase blood circulation.

— **Jin Shin Jyutsu** is a form of fully clothed massage that uses verbal guidance and light exercise. The major goal is to release chronic tension, referred to as "armoring," and rebalance your energy flow.

— **Kinesiology** (muscle testing) is based on the concept of internal energy fundamental to traditional Chinese medicine. Muscle testing is a noninvasive way of evaluating the body's imbalances and assessing its needs. It involves testing the body's responses when applying slight pressure to a large muscle to provide information on energy blockages, such as the functioning of the organs, nutritional deficiencies, and food sensitivities. It can also be used to test the body's responses to herbs and other remedies.

— **Lymph drainage** promotes a healthy lymphatic system. The lymphatic system is a complex network of tissues, organs, vessels, and ducts that moves bodily fluid. It helps filter toxins from blood as well as carry white blood cells called *lymphocytes* to tissues and organs when they're under attack.

— **Neurotherapy** is similar to biofeedback, as it involves altering neural events according to the new intent. This is helpful when wanting to let go of obsessive, unhealthy, or abusive thought patterns.

— **Pranic (energy) healing** is a highly evolved, intricate, and tested system of energy medicine that uses prana (energy) to balance, harmonize, and transform the body's energy. *Prana* is a Sanskrit word that means "life force." This invisible bioenergy keeps the body alive and helps it maintain a state of good health. It is also called *ruach* or the Breath of Life in Hebrew.

— **Reflexology** is a natural healing art based on the principle that there are reflexes in the feet, hands, and ears that correspond to every gland and organ of the body. Through application of pressure on these reflexes, you may relieve tension, improve circulation, and help promote the natural function of all areas of the body.

— **Shamanic healing** relies on the concept of luminescent energy fields that surround all material bodies. By meditating on both worlds, visible and invisible, shamans feel that they can heal themselves and others.

— **Shiatsu** is from *shi*, meaning "finger," and *atsu*, meaning "pressure." It's a traditional Japanese hands-on therapy based on anatomical and physiological theory and regulated as a licensed medical therapy in Japan. Pressure is applied to certain meridians and points in the body that help assist in moving stagnant *chi* or energy.

— **Therapeutic touch therapy** involves grounding and centering your whole being. With practice, you can bring the various aspects of your human energy field into total balance. The goal is to feel more at peace and focused as you become connected to your inner guides and teachers.

— **Traditional Chinese Medicine (TCM)** includes acupuncture, Chinese herbology, qigong, and Tui na—each of which offers a different way to balance and integrate your spirit, body, and mind. The underlying theory of TCM is that all beings and things in the universe have chi. When chi is abundant and flows freely, a natural state of balance and health prevails. When chi becomes excessive, deficient, or blocked, an energetic pattern is created that may lead to physical, emotional, mental, or spiritual problems.

The primary goal of Chinese medicine is to locate and correct imbalances in the circulation of chi. Imbalances may occur as a result of suppressed emotions, negative thought patterns, stress, physical trauma, poor diet, environmental factors, or unhealthy lifestyle choices.

Chinese medicine can be tailored to your unique situation. Treatment options include acupuncture, moxibustion, cupping, chi healing, and Chinese herbs. These are woven together to provide you with the best combination to restore or maintain the harmony of your spirit, mind, and body.

— **Vitamin infusions** are used to increase energy, decrease toxic stress, and increase the function of the body to do its job optimally. During this process, you receive an IV infusion with strong antioxidant and antiviral vitamins and minerals to help prevent illness, decrease stress, and increase energy.

You don't have to thoroughly possess the knowledge of any of these modalities in order for these systems of healing to work for you. Seek and you shall receive. Follow your intuition. Explore, have fun, be like a child, and be creative in your healing process. Don't stay stuck or negative. Learn something new. Expand your mind and soul by reaching out to find what works for *you*.

Next, we're going to look in depth at another critical component of healing: detoxification.

CHAPTER FOUR

Detox Time: Cleaning Inside and Out

Cleansing is as important as any procedure or modality to help support your healing that we've discussed so far. In fact, it's such an integral part of your health care that it deserves its own chapter. Note that there are many varieties of cleanses to suit individual needs, so I'm just going to talk about a few of my favorites here. I'll also guide you through the detoxification process itself and help you understand why it's so critical.

So far, you've had to reach outside yourself in an effort to find the help you need to kick cancer's ass. Now I'm asking you to dig deep, so to speak—you'll need to turn inward and flush out old stagnant toxins, emotions, and mind-sets. Our tendency is to hold on for dear life, especially when we're afraid. I'd like to inspire you to release in new ways as you go with the flow.

Detoxification Season

In Chinese medicine, every organ of the body correlates to a season. For example, spring is liver season. This is my favorite time of year—a time for new beginnings, rebirth, and renewal. It's liver time! In spring, the liver is like a flowering bulb coming up after the long winter months, ready to open, expand, and shake off its blanket of dirt.

After spring comes summer, the heart/small intestine season; fall, the lung/large intestine season; and then winter, the kidney/bladder season. Every organ also has its correlating emotion: the heart is all about joy, lungs express grief, kidneys are ruled by fear (fight or flight), the spleen is associated with sympathy, and the liver is affected by anger and frustration.

What does this mean? Well, if your liver filters your body's accumulation of toxins, then wouldn't it make sense that in its correlating season, it's ready to be detoxed? In other words, not only is spring a good time for your house to get a thorough cleaning, but it's a great season for internal cleansing as well. It is the ideal time to eliminate junk food, chemicals, and emotional and environmental toxins—but more specifically, it is in the spring that it is necessary for the liver to take a break from its heavy burdens.

Toxins must be cleared out of our temple/body at the opportune time. But how do we do this? One way is as old as the Bible. According to *The Essene Gospel of Peace,* which was translated and edited by Edmond Bordeaux Szekely, even Jesus speaks of cleaning out the body through colon irrigation, which is better known today as a "colonic" (more on this subject later in the chapter).

Another simple method of detoxification is to eliminate all toxic substances, such as: sugar or sugar substitutes; chemicals; fried food; gluten or wheat; dairy; alcohol; and drugs, including sleeping pills and caffeine. We feed our bodies only pure, organic foods and fluids. I also like to add in detoxing tools such as a shake or cleansing and healing herbs to get the most from my cleanse. It is more beneficial to do this at the right time, when the liver is ready, willing, and able.

Every spring, I lead groups of clients through a supported personalized cleanse. My favorite cleanses are those in which we gently detox the liver by consuming specific medicinal shakes and remedies, along with eating a more restricted diet of very clean foods. It's no accident that springtime is the season for a delicious array of fresh veggies and fruit. Temperatures warm up, so our bodies can handle the foods of the season—salads, raw juices, and locally grown fruits and vegetables.

In early spring, there is a period I call "pre-cleanse." As you begin the process, you may notice a rash or breakout with various kinds of skin eruptions. You might have discharge through the eyes with pinkeye or some eye twitching. Whenever I ask my groups of detoxers, "Whose eyes have been mysteriously twitching?" it never fails—more than half the hands in the crowd go up. The pre-cleanse period is the liver's way of saying, "Hello, welcome to the season . . . now get to work and clean me, please."

I've heard of women detoxing their livers in the middle of winter with a five- or even ten-day "Master Cleanse" that consists of living on a drink made with hot water, lemon, cayenne, and maple syrup. I don't agree with this protocol because winter is not the natural time to detox the liver—such a cleanse depletes us when we need to build, sustain, ground, and hunker down. If someone feels the need to drink only warm, nourishing fluids for a period of 24 to 48 hours, or as a supplement to a cleaner diet, it can be beneficial. In the frigid temperatures of winter, I suggest adding warming herbs such as turmeric, ginger, and cayenne.

Winter is a time for hearty stews and soups with root veggies. Doesn't that sound much better than a cold salad with raw veggies and a frozen-fruit smoothie? Winter is a time to pull inward and hunker down, in preparation for hibernation. It is a time for reflection.

Picture a daffodil or tulip: It starts as a seedling hiding under a warm blanket of dirt all winter long, gathering strength from the nutrient-rich soil. In spring, it pushes up through the dirt into a new day, and the sunshine warms and the rain hydrates this baby plant. Human beings are very similar to plants in that we also need to gather nutrients and stay grounded over the winter. When spring comes, we are rejuvenated and ready to shake off "the dirt" as we reach taller toward the sun. This is when we're ready to drink the wheatgrass juice, eat the salads, and enjoy the veggies and fruits of spring and summer. Ah, doesn't the idea of a cleanse sound much better now?

Detoxification Reason

I don't want to overwhelm you or make you paranoid, but here's another great reason to cleanse: we're all being pummeled by thousands of toxic metals and compounds every day. The air we breathe, the foods we eat, and the water we drink and bathe in are all contaminated.

You need look no further than Dr. David Servan-Schreiber's book *Anticancer: A New Way of Life,* in which he cites studies conducted by scientists, researchers, and all manner of brilliant people regarding the sheer amount of chemicals we're exposed to on a daily basis. It's truly mind-boggling. When you see the study about children tested for pesticide residue, it will make you sick. This book is well worth reading . . . but be prepared, you will want to take out a Brillo pad and scrub your body inside and out.

Studies indicate that we have between 400 and 800 toxic metal and chemical residues stored in our bodies. They accumulate in our fat cells; breast tissue; bones; major organs, such as the liver, kidneys, and brain; and glands, such as the thyroid and adrenals. And, according to the website **Evenbetterhealth.com**: "There are 34,000 pesticides and herbicides registered with the Environmental Protection Agency (EPA). . . . Over one-fourth of the four billion pounds of pesticides used in the world are used in the United States. Each year, 10,000 chemicals are being synthesized by industry and added to the over one million already in existence."

Virtually all of us are now in a state of overload from environmental toxins commonly found in shampoo, soap, perfume, deodorant, prescription drugs, vaccines, hair dye, newspapers, dry cleaning, exhaust fumes, carpets, cleaning products, paints, solvents, glues, herbicides, pesticides, and fertilizers. This chemical buildup hinders our body's ability to function, making it unable to assimilate and utilize essential minerals such as iron, calcium, and magnesium.

EPA scientists have concluded that the total toxic residue in our daily diet can exceed 500 percent of the recommended daily maximum—I don't know about you, but this is unacceptable for me. I want to be proactive and do whatever I can to protect myself, so I cleanse.

Detoxification Cleanses

Cleanses have become the biggest fad since aerobics with Jane Fonda. Even so, they shouldn't be taken lightly. As a cancer patient, or as a survivor, the question of when to cleanse goes beyond the time of the year.

First, it really should be done under the supervision of a professional, especially if you're a first-time detoxer. I have seen some products being sold as part of a detox program that are full of junk. I mean it—they're loaded with sugar and a long list of chemicals, preservatives, and just plain empty calories. It's sad to think that people are having their detox hopes and dreams shattered by these inferior and sometimes dangerous products.

Second, if you have cancer and are currently undergoing any kind of treatment, cleanses are not for you at this time. Unfortunately, most of the harsh chemicals used in chemotherapy regimens should not be cleansed out of the liver in the middle of your treatment. And if you feel weak, dehydrated, or depleted, detoxing could exacerbate these physical symptoms.

I like to finish all treatments, then rebuild and strengthen my immune system by eating clean, good-quality whole foods and beverages (as I describe in detail in Chapter 5). So before *you* start any sort of detox, make sure that you're strong enough in terms of overall health, weight, and energy level.

When you're ready, here are some tips to keep in mind:

- Again, I want to stress that if you're in the middle of harsh treatments, wait until you're finished, and rebuild first.

- Note that the detox should be at least 28 days in length to fully cleanse your liver.

- Find a trusted health-care professional who offers high-quality options.

- Give the liver and colon a head start by having a good colonic.

- Find a product with organic ingredients so you know it isn't biochemically engineered and is chemical free. Make sure the sugar content is low, and there's no high-fructose corn syrup, soy protein isolate, or other preservatives or additives.

- Look for at least 15 grams of pure protein per serving from organic whey or rice.

- Be sure to incorporate clean, organic foods into your diet.

I never limit myself to only one method of detox. And when it comes to my clients, I like to mix a variety of cleansing techniques depending upon each person's unique physical condition, environment, and history. I've detailed a few of my favorites in the pages that follow.

Metagenics Cleanse

Metagenics is a company I have worked with for more than 20 years. I trust them with all of my clients' detoxing needs, as well as my own. Specific Metagenics detoxification programs provide macro- and micronutrients in greater concentrations than is found in some commercial products.

All Metagenics cleanses come with a step-by-step guide that incorporates specific guidelines to enhance gentle phase II liver detoxification, and each of them is uniquely designed to address a person's physical symptoms. (For example, their UltraClear Plus pH aids in balancing the body's pH by alkalinizing through the bloodstream and urine.) So, since each cleanse is as unique as a person's biochemical makeup, everyone can expect to feel something different on these cleanses. (Do note that some people experience headaches, sweats, and dizziness.)

After the initial detox phase, my clients start to experience increased energy, as well as thinking and seeing things from a clearer perspective. A common remark I get from first-time cleansers is, "I feel like I have bionic vision and hearing now."

Clay Cleanse

One of the most effective and inexpensive means of pulling all kinds of chemicals and heavy metals out of the body is through clay. The best one for detoxification is Bentonite clay, or calcium montmorillonite. It is also known as "living clay," for it consists of highly absorbable minerals that enhance the production of enzymes in all living organisms. You can use it in a bath, or make it into a mudpack by adding water. If you try this option, be like a kid finger painting and have a ball painting your belly and upper rib cage. Then, rest in the sun for about 20 minutes.

You can find clay at your local health-food stores or online. I like to keep it on hand for all emergencies, such as bee or wasp stings. It pulls the poison right out and alleviates the pain of the sting. You can also use it for a wound that won't stop bleeding or even for food poisoning. Clay does effectively remove toxins from the body when taken internally. However, since there's a variety available for internal use, please see your health-care practitioner for instructions.

Vitamin-Infusion Cleanse

Vitamin infusions are great cleanses. These can be done as a form of high-dose vitamin C therapy, or you can add a variety of other essential vitamins and minerals.

Vitamin C is one of the most common vitamin deficiencies seen today, especially for those undergoing chemotherapy—yet our ability to neutralize the effects of pollutants depends upon our daily intake of it. Ascorbates found in this vitamin are also very effective detoxifiers of heavy metals and chemical poisons. They aid in ridding the body of lead, mercury, carbon monoxide, sulfur dioxide, various carcinogens, bacterial toxins, and poisons; and they protect us from benzene exposure.

If you eat an all-raw-food diet of freshly picked and naturally ripened fruits and vegetables, as well as sprouted seeds and grains, you're most likely to give your body the amount of vitamin C and other minerals it needs daily. This is doable if you live on a farm. If you live in a city or in a colder climate, your body's daily vitamin C requirements are going to be much higher, due to the toxic exposure of urban living and lack of sufficient fresh produce.

If you do happen to live where it's cold, it is not immune-efficient to live on raw food all winter long. Doing so can cause you to lose much of your body's heat, which you need to help keep you insulated. I know this firsthand because I live in Chicago. I would simply wither up and die on a raw-food diet in the middle of this city's brutal winter months.

It is an absolute must to get a baseline idea of what vitamins and minerals you're depleted in as you go through treatments of any kind. I suggest that you request your heavy-metal levels as well. Your hospital will test you for anything you ask for, and insurance will usually cover it. You can request testing for your levels of vitamins D and E, calcium, and magnesium, too. And have all your hormone levels tested while you're at it, so you can get a good base. Then take those results to a natural practitioner you trust to explain them to you. This person can also help you find ways to replenish your body with the necessary minerals, nutrients, and vitamins it needs.

When I asked one of my "regular" doctors about my own levels, he seemed to think everything was acceptable. Kind of like how it's acceptable to have certain amounts of arsenic in our public water system. When I took the results to my natural doctor, though, he explained how my heavy-metal levels were high; and I was depleted in other areas, including vitamin D and magnesium. For me, vitamin infusions were the answer—after only one year, I cut my high mercury levels in half. I've continued doing them ever since.

Herbs that Cleanse

As we know, the liver is the main organ of detoxification and needs to be supported when undergoing any regimen to remove heavy metals and toxins. God has given us amazing herbs that aid in detoxification while feeding/healing our organs. For example, algin (derived from seaweeds such as kelp and dulse) and algae (such as chlorella) provide protection from many of today's pollutants, and kelp has been shown to block certain heavy metals from being absorbed by the body.

A great way to detox heavy metals is by using sodium alginate (an extract of kelp) and apple pectin. Take 1,000 mg of sodium alginate and/or 500 mg of apple pectin per day for every 100 pounds of body weight, for at least 12 weeks (or much longer for severe metal toxicity).

Cleansing herbs can also help people recover from a buildup of pharmaceutical drugs and environmental toxins. These herbs are right out of a Harry Potter movie, with names like bugleweed, yellow dock, and lobelia. One of my favorite herbs, chaparral, is an extremely potent blood purifier and can be drunk as a tea: Put ¼ tsp. of loose-leaf chaparral in a 10-oz. cup of hot water, then steep for three minutes, and strain through a tea strainer. It can be tough to swallow due to its bitter taste, so drink up fast. Don't let it stand too long.

Another great detoxifying remedy is cilantro paste, which has been proven to chelate toxic metals from our bodies effectively and quickly. Thank goodness, this one actually tastes great:

CILANTRO CHELATION HEAVY-METAL CLEANSE

Combine the following and drink:

4 cloves garlic

⅓ cup Brazil nuts (selenium source)

⅓ cup sunflower seeds (cysteine source)

⅓ cup pumpkin seeds (zinc, magnesium sources)

2 cups packed fresh cilantro—or coriander or
  Chinese parsley (vitamin A source)
⅔ cup flaxseed oil
4 Tbsp. lemon juice (vitamin C source)
2 tsp. dulse powder
Bragg Liquid Aminos

Salt Cleanse

Taking a bath in the evening with three to six cups of Epsom salts and one to three cups of baking soda is a great way to pull toxins from the physical body. Speaking of baking soda (or sodium bicarbonate), there is a whole movement of natural practitioners suggesting that we drink it for its alkalinizing/cleansing properties—they feel it aids in the body's ability to eliminate the fungus, mold, and yeast that are contributing factors to cancer. I drink it, and it actually works! Google "baking soda and cancer" for some interesting facts.

As far as salt goes, I'd like to inspire you to be creative when using it for its healing properties. Have some fun by making your own concoction to use as a scrub on your skin in the shower—I mix Himalayan pink salt with honey and coconut oil, for instance. If you search online, you'll find a plethora of available scrubs. Some websites will even tell you how to make your own creation by combining emollient and essential oils, mud, charcoal, or herbs. By the time you're done, you might feel like a basted turkey, but you'll be clean!

Whether you're soaking or scrubbing, remember that the detoxifying properties in salt are far reaching, and your skin will look great, too.

Enema Cleanse

Your large intestine is a hollow, tubelike organ that moves toxic materials along by wavelike motions called peristaltic action. Constipation can be caused by a variety of things, including not immediately responding to the "call of nature," not eating a sufficient amount of greens, and dehydration.

The natural immune system can only run at peak performance in a clean body; that is, one with a minimal amount of accumulated toxic material. If the large intestine is infested with harmful bacteria and parasites, this may contribute to more serious diseases—such as cancer—in the long run.

Parasites may be defined as any living organisms that live on or in another living organism. Signs of parasite infection include constipation, diarrhea, gas, bloating, abdominal pain, nausea, vomiting, rash or itching around the rectum, and weight loss. International travel, poor-quality food or water, poor hygiene, and a weakened immune system can all contribute to the presence of parasites.

When "parasites" are mentioned to doctors, they typically think of worms, but molds and fungi are also classified in this way. After all, if food is left out or remains too long in the refrigerator, it will start to develop mold: the outcome is parasitic in nature.

If you're going through chemotherapy, you run the risk of contracting parasites because your intestinal tract is depleted of good bacteria. Therefore, you must make sure that the food you eat is fresh and of the highest quality (taking a good probiotic will help, too).

Parasites can be eliminated through deep cleansing, with either a colon irrigation done by a professional or a home enema. Using herbs such as wormwood and black walnut to rid the body of parasites is very effective—be it orally or infused into your intestines by way of an enema bag—but if you're undergoing treatments of any kind, consult a qualified practitioner before you take these herbs.

The most valuable gift I gave myself was learning how to administer a home enema. Some people are under the misconception that enemas can hurt you or may not be healthy, but they couldn't be more wrong. Enemas are a great way to make sure that you're cleaning out the waste from your body every day. I know many people might be embarrassed when it comes to this delicate and private matter, but proper elimination is essential. It is necessary to cleanse the liver, gut, intestines, and bowel of all the toxicity that chemotherapy, drugs from surgeries, and radiation can cause.

Sometimes I use coffee enemas to detoxify my liver. Yes, coffee is a stimulant, but I'm not recommending you drink it. Instead, I'm suggesting that you cleanse with it! This type of enema goes directly into the toxic liver and helps release the buildup of chemicals and sludge. Needless to say, most people tend to be nervous about inserting a tube that releases coffee into their rectum. I can empathize. I will only say that once you feel the amazing benefits from it, you will love it. Once you jump-start the colon, it will work more efficiently, and you will feel so much lighter and free.

To perform a coffee enema, you'll need an enema bag from your local pharmacy. Once you've read the directions, take ½ cup or so of organic ground coffee in any flavor. Jamaican, French, or Mexican—have fun choosing, especially if you're not able to drink it.

Boil the coffee of your choice in about 4 cups of water. Let it cool down, making sure it's at room temperature. (If you're in a hurry, you can mix it with some cold water.) Then strain the coffee with a metal mesh strainer into a large glass beaker or measuring cup. Don't use plastic, since it leaches toxic residue.

Pour the coffee into the enema bag. Make yourself comfortable by lying on some old towels and place a pillow under your head. Take your time. Lie on your right side so the coffee will go right into your liver, which is on your right side under your breast. You can control how much you let into your rectum with a clamp that comes with the enema bag. Let a little in at a time until you feel the need to release your bowels. Then get up and calmly walk over to the toilet. Don't worry . . . you will not lose control of your bowels.

Make sure you have plenty of magazines on hand, as you will repeat this process about three to four times until the liquid in your enema bag is gone. Don't cheat yourself out of the whole bag of liquid, because it takes that much to get the maximum release.

I promise you will feel great!

When deciding to enema or not to enema, keep in mind that one study showed that women who have two or fewer bowel movements per week have four times the risk of breast disease as women who have one or more per day.

I love to talk about poop; it's one of my favorite subjects (besides food, of course). I actually have had poop envy on many occasions. There is a cute little book called *What's Your Poo Telling You?* It teaches that the normal color of a stool is golden honey brown, with minimal offensive odor. If your poops are really dark, look for signs and symptoms such as allergies, bad breath, depression, skin problems, hemorrhoids, and any other digestive issues. If you have rabbit turds, this means you're dehydrated. Small, hard poops can also occur when you go through your scans because the contrast they make you swallow is dehydrating. Please drink a ton of fluids whenever you're done with a scan, treatment, or surgery.

The final word on poop: It is supposed to follow the shape of your intestines. It should look like a snake, long and curled around the toilet bowl. When you're lucky enough to create a poop you like, you may feel some sort of pride. You'll want to show it off to your family members. What? No one's home? Then quick, go get a neighbor!

Colon Hydrotherapy Cleanse

A colonic will work on a deeper level than a home enema because it goes higher into the upper gastrointestinal (GI) tract. I don't like the new high-pressure colonics that are out there now; I like the old-fashioned gravity method.

I suggest finding someone you trust to give you a colonic. I go to a wonderful, loving woman named Alyce at Partners in Wellness in the Chicago area. I have cried through many a session as I let go of not only physical poop but emotional poop as well. I go for it—I let it all hang out. I love Alyce because she's kind and gentle, and she uses oils to massage my belly and relax me, as well as techniques to help me release. She adds chlorophyll and/or acidophilus powder to the water, helping me build the good bacteria in my gut. If I feel I might have a parasite, she'll add woodworm and/or black walnut to the water.

I once went to a colonic Nazi in Florida who scared the shit out of me, literally. She was amazing, but she was so intense I couldn't go to her anymore. If you ever have a not-so-great experience, don't let that ruin things for you and your toxins. Quit your whining and go find another practitioner.

Emotional Cleanse

Cleansing is not just about the physical self—it's about your *emotional* self as well. I've noticed both personally and with my clients that during spring, we can feel overwhelmed with emotions, which may be old and stagnant. My suggestion is that we don't stuff our feelings; rather, we need to dig deep and bless our bodies for working. In order to move forward, we must let the past go.

Here are some tips to help you through what I call an "emotional cleansing":

— Make a list of all your grudges, frustrations, dislikes, and grievances. Then create a meditation around them such as the Buddhist "loving-kindness meditation" (I like Pema Chödrön's version). Or, create your very own loving-kindness ritual or chant and picture forgiving all the people who have hurt you.

Let them go with love and send them off in a bubble of white light. I like to shrink whoever has hurt me in my hand, in the bubble of white light, and then gently blow

73

them away as I set them free. There they go, floating away in their own protected space. . . .

— Write down all the dreams you have stored away and put on a shelf somewhere, then mark them off your list as you accomplish them one by one.

— Create a sacred space inside or out—then every morning or evening, perform a cleansing ritual for your emotional healing. I like to go into my yoga space, strip off all my clothing, and meditate in the nude, as if somehow I'm being baptized or bathed in light as I breathe and wash away the emotional baggage from the past.

— Find a space where you can reconnect to the light, your source, or whatever your higher power is; feel yourself enveloped in self-love and acceptance. Realize your purpose as you sit quietly day after day. Plant the seeds of perfect health as you meditate on your healthy body, heart, and mind. Forgive yourself in this sacred space, and make amends with yourself and others.

Dig in deep as you clean away all the muck. Cry, laugh, and hug yourself. Get to know your beautiful new body with all its new scars, if that's the case. When we're naked, we feel liberated and free, and we gain a sense of what our bodies really feel and look like. No shame, no guilt, no judgment—just look at your body as the beautiful gift it is.

— When I absolutely must rid myself of negative emotional ties or something that I just can't seem to shake loose, I burn it in a ceremony. The full moon is a powerful time to ask the universe to help you let go, and the new moon is a great time for bringing in our desires. I write or draw a picture of the thing I must eliminate from my life and then create a ceremony around it as I burn it. I watch the ashes fly away as the problem goes with it, into the winds.

— Finally, try the Native American technique that's known as a "tree giveaway." Take a personal belonging that is reminiscent of your problem, and then wrap it in a piece of fabric with some coffee beans or corn kernels as an offering to the earth. Hang your giveaway on a tree, and say a prayer as you let go of all the items in the bag. (No, you cannot hang an industrial-size garbage bag with all your problems from the neighbor's tree.)

More options are available for cleansing than those I've listed here; in fact, there are as many varieties of cleanses as there are people who need a good cleanse.

Cleansing is absolutely necessary for healing. After you've let go both physically and emotionally, you'll see things more clearly, as if you've awakened from a sort of slumber. You will feel acutely alive. Celebrate like it's your birthday, for you have been reborn.

CHAPTER FIVE

Let Food Be Thy Medicine

After you do a cleanse, you might discover that some of the foods you've been living on don't actually make you feel very good. You could feel so inspired that you find that you don't want to go back to the old crap; cleanses can be quite motivating.

Now that you've read all about my love of detoxing, you may not guess that my favorite subject is food. I *love* to eat—it's the priority of my life. I also enjoy teaching others that a healthful diet is the number one line of defense against any disease. I hear the same questions over and over again: "What do you eat?" and "How are you able to eat so well?" This chapter contains my answers.

Food can be our medicine or our poison. Processed foods, alcohol, caffeine, sugar, and poor-quality fats are detrimental to every aspect of our health. Healing foods are not frozen or canned; they are not leftovers saved in the refrigerator for more than two days.

Rather, they consist of fresh grains, beans and other legumes, vegetables, fruits, and possibly small amounts of good-quality animal protein.

I recently came across a photographic essay that asked families from all around the world to display one week's worth of meals for their family on a table. Families from most countries, particularly less developed ones, displayed foods indigenous to their region, such as: whole grains, beans and legumes, fresh fruits and vegetables, meat, poultry, and eggs; with a small amount of packaged or processed foods. Of course, the American table overflowed with brightly colored packaged items—only about 20 percent consisted of foods that came from nature. And we wonder why this country is in a health crisis! Why are cancer, diabetes, heart disease, autoimmune disorders, and neurological diseases at epidemic proportions? Welcome to the USA.

I can't believe the crap some Americans are living on . . . but in this country, processed food is big business. Many European countries have refused to allow the bio-chemically engineered seeds or products that we consume every day into their market because studies have shown that this type of processing can be detrimental to one's health. They're choosing to protect their people, while our nation ransoms its inhabitants' well-being to promote the corporate bottom line. Our great country still refuses to place the label "GMO" on products that contain genetically modified ingredients. I personally believe, and have witnessed, that food can hurt or heal. I wish the American medical profession would offer this component of health care, or at least not pooh-pooh it.

This brings to mind the time I brought Michio Kushi's *The Cancer Prevention Diet* to a client in the hospital who was fighting breast cancer. This eye-opening book is one of my favorites, and I like to give it to many of my clients because it is very easy to use. You simply look up the type of cancer you're dealing with, and it gives you specific reasons for how you got it. The best parts of this clever guide are its in-depth suggestions of what you can do now to make healthy, alternative changes.

My client was devouring the book, as I knew she would, when an old-school doctor came into her room with a group of medical students. "See this book?" he told them, as he rudely grabbed it out of her hand. "This is a huge waste of time." How sad.

Dena's Do's and Don'ts of Cancer

I have witnessed people go into remission after adopting a macrobiotic lifestyle, or one that's similar in nature. I happen to love macrobiotic food and how it makes me feel, so I didn't find it all that difficult to change my way of life. But others *do* find the change difficult, since such a diet can be limiting and feel aggressive for most Westerners—many of whom are addicted to caffeine, meat, and sugar. When it comes to saving your life, it's certainly worth looking into.

On the next few pages, I share the eating program I've developed, which is a bit more palatable for Westerners than a strict macrobiotic diet. I never call what I've created for others or myself a "diet"—it is simply a beautiful and health-promoting way of life, which helped me kick cancer's ass and can do the same for you.

First, I'll talk about the items you should eliminate or limit. But don't despair . . . when you see all that you get to incorporate into your life, and experience how great they'll make you feel, you won't feel as if you're being asked to give up anything. You will actually feel so much better on so many levels—physically, mentally, and emotionally—that you will become addicted to your new food. (Note that you may want to recruit a member of your support team to help you meet your daily responsibilities of shopping and cooking nutritious foods for yourself. Enlisting a friend or family member to join you on this journey will make it fun!)

— **Don't eat sugar.** Getting off sugar is no easy task, as most of us are addicted to it, and for good reason—it is in almost everything we eat, from candy to ketchup. Yet sugar attacks the immune system, causes inflammation, and is dehydrating (and we're already dehydrated from treatments). It also adds unnecessary stress and burden to the kidneys, which are the filtration system for the body, and the adrenal glands. And it fuels and feeds cancer. *You read me right . . . sugar, including the natural sugar found in fruit, can contribute to the growth of cancer in your body.*

You probably don't even realize how many everyday symptoms come from a sugar-filled diet: mood swings, fatigue, sleep issues, compulsivity, ADD, depression, anger, and frustration, to name a few. (A great book to read about all this is *Sugar Blues* by William Dufty.) As you wean yourself from that seductive substance, you may experience some or all of the following: headaches or light-headedness, crabbiness (including anger and frustration), fatigue, and even nausea. These withdrawal symptoms will pass after about three days, and you will feel clearer and have more energy. Even your appearance will be different.

Yes, you will feel as if you need an exorcist as you're coming off of sugar. But I promise that you will feel amazing once you quit. I'll never forget what it felt like after the "wanting to murder someone" stage passed for me. Everything became crystal clear—the fog had lifted—and I was naturally high.

Note: I'm not saying you can't eat sugar ever again. After the cancer was in remission, I felt I could treat myself to some fruit-juice-sweetened goodies. So I made Jam-Dot Cookies, using organic, fruit-juice-sweetened jam and a bit of brown-rice syrup. They were so yummy, and they hit the sugar spot. (The recipe is in my cookbook, which is available on my website.)

— **Don't use sugar substitutes.** Some of these are actually worse than sugar; in fact, if you Google many sugar substitutes, you'll see that they're dangerous, if not downright deadly. Take, for example, aspartame (or NutraSweet). Found in diet soft drinks and many other sugar-free foods, including the gum our kids chew, aspartame is a known neurotoxin—it can cause migraines, dizziness, sleep disorders, and weight gain. Also, stay away from saccharin (or Sweet'N Low) and sucralose (or Splenda). My motto is: "Eat the real deal."

— **Don't eat processed grains.** I once heard Madonna say that white sugar is the devil, and white flour is its brother. But whole wheat is not much better. In fact, all wheat products wreak havoc in our lives by stressing our immune systems. I see a definite connection among my clients with inflammatory issues such as cancer and an overconsumption of wheat—but, in actuality, *no one* does well on a diet loaded with processed carbs.

— **Don't eat gluten.** Many people don't even know what gluten is, so I'll give you a quick overview. *Gluten* is a protein derivative of wheat, rye, barley, and oats; the dictionary describes it as a substance that gives dough "a more elastic character." I say that gluten resembles glue or sludge in the gut, sinuses, and other organs.

Eliminating gluten from your diet means avoiding wheat, rye, and most oats—this means cookies, crackers, pasta, cake, muffins, pastries, and pizza crust. At first, this list might seem extremely restrictive, but with so many people allergic to wheat and gluten today, many wonderful alternatives exist. There's no need to suffer or feel deprived.

Check the label on the product to make sure that it says "No wheat" and "No gluten." Make sure that your choices don't have too much sugar—sometimes a product compensates for a lack of wheat by adding sugar. The trick with most wheat- and gluten-free bread is that it must be toasted. (You can find hints like this in my cookbook, which features gluten-free recipes.)

I do not recommend most "meat substitutes." Most faux meat products, which can be found in the freezer section, contain wheat and gluten as their number one ingredient. If you enjoy an occasional veggie sausage in your wheat- and gluten-free pasta (Tinkyada is the best brand for pasta), then go ahead. I wouldn't live on processed packaged products as staples, though, as they're not beneficial for us. God certainly didn't intend for us to eat food out of a box. We are looking to *live*, so we want to eat *live* foods that will sustain us.

— **Don't eat dairy products.** Many people don't understand all that dairy encompasses. For example, a woman came to me once with a terrible case of burning in her stomach. I took her off caffeine, wheat and gluten, and dairy. She was feeling much better after we weaned her off all inflammatory foods and acid-promoting beverages such as soda. Then one day she called me and said that she wasn't sure why she still had a tiny amount of burning. I had a feeling I would find the culprit in her kitchen, so I went over to investigate.

As I was looking through her refrigerator, I noticed a sea of yogurt. And not the sugar-filled Yoplait-type that so many women are into, but the really high-quality Greek kind. I asked her who ate so much yogurt, and she innocently replied, "It's for me. I eat it every morning." I laughed and told her that I thought we'd agreed on no dairy. She looked at me and said, "Oh, is that dairy?" I said, "No, it's meat."

This one funny girl made me realize that sometimes even highly intelligent people think that because something is high in quality, it is somehow exempt from causing pain and suffering. Dairy products do cause inflammation, which can promote cancer—so no milk, cheese, ice cream, yogurt, or sour cream while you're fighting this fight. (No, eggs are not dairy; they are a good source of protein, however, and I talk more about them in the "Do" section.)

— **Don't ingest any alcohol or caffeine.** These substances undermine immune response, are toxic and dehydrating, and slow down your metabolism. Your body already has to process enough chemicals without adding more to the mix. Keep picturing it as your temple, and visualize all the wonderfully healthy things you want to put into it. The rule of thumb I follow is to never put any fluids into my body that are murky or brown in color (such as soda, coffee, milk, shakes, or fruit juice).

— **Don't use microwave ovens.** I have a funny story about microwaves. I was going to heat up some food for a 15-year-old client, so I took out a frying pan and a pot. She asked, "Why don't you use a microwave?" I told her more than she cared to know about why you should never use a microwave. Then she very casually asked, "How do you make a hot dog?" I had to laugh. She had no idea you could make a grass-fed, organic hot dog in a boiling pot of water, toaster oven, or grill.

As the August 16, 2006, issue of the Harvard Medical School e-newsletter HEALTHbeat (**www.health .harvard.edu/healthbeat/HEALTHbeat_081606.htm**) noted: "When food is wrapped in plastic or placed in a plastic container and microwaved, substances used in manufacturing the plastic (plasticizers) may leak into the food. In particular, fatty foods such as meats and cheeses cause a chemical called diethylhexyl adipate to leach out."

I don't even own a microwave oven because I believe that such devices deplete the nutrients in food. (Of course, any heating of food may result in a loss of nutrients.) I don't even want to stand near one when it's on, especially after reading the "Effects of Microwave Radiation on Anti-infective Factors in Human Milk," by researchers at Stanford University. This clinical study, published in *Pediatrics*, discovered that microwaving breast milk at high temperatures caused a marked decrease in activity of all the tested anti-infective factors. They found that microwave radiation led to a significant loss of the immunological properties of milk; thus, they concluded that microwaving is definitely "not a suitable heat treatment modality for breast milk." In their abstract, the Stanford researchers noted: "Microwaving appears to be contraindicated at high temperatures, and questions regarding its safety exist even at low temperatures." That's evidence enough for me.

— **Don't eat mucus-causing foods.** *Mucus* is another word for *phlegm*. Normal phlegm is a necessary substance in terms of our mucous membrane lining, and it aids in lubricating bodily functions. Mucus becomes a pathological substance only when it's derived from stagnated food in the stomach, or if we can't digest or break down the poor-quality foods we are consuming, which in turn makes it difficult to eliminate. If this mucuslike substance is produced in excess and then stagnates, it becomes too much for our body to process, thereby becoming toxic. When our digestive tract is sluggish or inefficient, it prevents phlegm from being eliminated. When this happens, there is congestion, which will create a host of problems in the sinuses, lungs, and bowels. It can even cause adipose (fat) accumulation.

As we know, cancer is an inflammatory disorder, and one primary indication of this is the physical presence of mucus. In fact, tumors that have been removed are most often encased in mucus, like mine was. Foods that contribute to a large amount of phlegm are all found on my "Don'ts" list.

— **Don't eat poor-quality animal fats.** I'm an O blood type, so I can eat as much animal protein as I like, according to *Eat Right 4 Your Type*. This book, by Dr. Peter J. D'Adamo, professes that there is a specific diet for each blood type and even suggests what people can and can't digest according to their particular type.

I had an Asian friend who was chunky and couldn't seem to lose weight. She was also tired all the time. I asked her what blood type she was over dinner one night. As she sat there chomping away at her porterhouse, she told me she was an A blood type. "Aha," I retorted, "vegetarian. No wonder you are tired and have bad breath all the time, along with terrible psoriasis. Not a good combo." She went off all meat, and lo and behold, all her problems seemed to magically disappear. She told me later that she really didn't even like meat.

I myself don't follow any one particular "diet." First and foremost, I do what feels right for me under specific circumstances, such as the season or how I'm feeling according to treatments. If my digestion feels sluggish and gives me clues—such as hiccups, indigestion, or constipation—I won't consume foods that would burden my already-compromised digestion and liver, like heavy concentrations of beef. I don't care what anyone says: when my organs are under stress, I know, without a doubt, that I should not eat meat. I often choose other, more easily digestible proteins—such as beans, legumes, and fish. But when I *am* ready for a small amount of protein, I make sure it is of the highest quality.

Once again, I say, "Know thyself." Get to know who you are and how your body feels after everything you eat. How does meat make you feel? Also, when treating yourself to small quantities of animal fats, remember this: when our ancestors ate beef, it came from cows that roamed free and ate grass. Today, most of our beef comes from cattle fed a diet of grains that have been treated with pesticides or that are biochemically engineered. Cows are also fed hormones to ensure maximum growth.

I prefer to eat beef from cattle that have roamed fields, eaten alkaline grass, and been treated humanely. We can debate whether or not the cattle is healthier from this more organic and humane lifestyle until, well, the cows come home—but I know I feel much better consuming grass-fed organic beef.

On an emotional level, I also believe that eating the meat of animals that have been mistreated is unhealthy. Check out John Robbins's classic, *Diet for a New America*. Once you've read about angry chickens penned tightly together in small cages suffocated by the looming smell of death, you may think twice about digesting that negative energy.

Don't get me wrong; I'm not saying you should never eat meat. The key is to buy free-range, organic, and/or grass-fed options if you're going to indulge. You must also assess your own digestive system. I most often choose wild-caught deep-sea fish for my protein. Test this concept out for yourself and see if you feel better eating less animal protein while you're supporting your digestive tract through the chemotherapy process, and even for a few months to a year afterward.

●○●

— **Do eat like your ancestors.** Eating seasonally, along with choosing locally grown food whenever possible, is best for your body. What grows in nature from trees and bushes will always promote life. So put down the packaged pretzels and go for the carrots. Cooking and eating healthier foods may take more time than just opening a box or ordering takeout, but you're worth it, right? After all, your body is your temple, so the food you give it should be pristine.

People ask me, "What diet would you put me on?" Yet there is no "one size fits all" diet. Everyone requires a specific way of life that suits their particular needs according to their health challenges and the environment they live in. But for anyone with life-threatening illnesses like cancer, I strongly recommend an eating plan that consists of whole, noninflammatory grains; vegetables, including sea vegetables such as seaweed (more on that later in the chapter); beans and legumes; and small amounts of protein from fish.

Clients often ask me about eggs. I like them and feel that they're an easily digestible protein, especially when they're organic from free-range hens. Again, see how you feel, but I like having eggs about once or twice a week. While I was going through chemotherapy, I wasn't eating meat, so I definitely enjoyed my eggs. Since the cancer I had was not estrogen receptive, I also ate tofu—but if the cancer you have *is* estrogen positive, limit your soy to very little, if any. In that case, free-range eggs would be an excellent choice for you.

When you make yourself a delicious and healthy plate of food, be sure to make it a fanciful display. I like to create a beautiful-looking meal fit for a queen. And always give yourself the time to sit, breathe, and chew well. Taking the time to enjoy your food will help your digestion *and* your mind-set . . . both of which increase the healing.

— **Do eat greens, greens, and more greens.** The darker the green, the more nutrient rich it is. The top superfoods are, in order: collard greens, mustard greens, turnip greens, kale, watercress, bok choy, spinach, brussels sprouts, Swiss chard, arugula, radish, and cabbage. The more greens you eat, the more alkaline your body will be. I'll choose alkaline green food over a more acidic meat dish any day (I talk more about alkalinity and acidity in just a bit). When I do eat some good-quality meat, I surround that amount with three times as many greens.

While the USDA recommends eating at least five servings of fruits and vegetables a day, I'd like to "one-up" the government and insist that they be organic. Eating organic fruits and vegetables minimizes the toxic effect of pesticide/herbicide ingestion. Also, keep the following charts in mind when shopping for produce:

Produce with the highest levels of pesticide residue	
Strawberries	Bell peppers
Celery	Spinach
Peaches	Cherries
Apples	Kale/collards
All berries	Potatoes
Nectarines	Grapes

Produce with the lowest levels of pesticide residue	
Onions	Eggplant
Avocados	Cantaloupe
Pineapple	Watermelon
Mangoes	Grapefruit
Asparagus	Sweet potatoes
Kiwi	Honeydew melons
Cabbage	

Wash all fruits and vegetables before eating. Even if washing doesn't completely eliminate pesticide residue, it sure does help. Peeling can help, too; but when in doubt, buy organic.

— **Do limit your fruit.** Yes, you should limit fruit for the time being. This won't be forever, but for now you must get off all sugar, and that includes the natural sugar found in fruits.

Throughout this guide, I recommend eating locally grown, seasonal, and organic fruit—as long as you're not coming from an extremely immune-deficient place. If you're in remission, you may add back some local, seasonal, low-sugar fruits such as berries or cherries. Tropical fruits such as pineapple, bananas, and mangoes are too high in sugar. I personally eat very little fruit, and only in warm weather. Remember, our goal is to *starve* cancer.

Alkalinity vs. Acidity

Think of your body as a garden—you want to cultivate the healthiest possible terrain and soil for it to grow. According to many experts, the healthiest environment for the body is one in which its cells are properly oxygenated, and its fluids and tissues have a balanced pH. When the body is too acidic or too alkaline, it will slow down in enzyme activity and cellular repair.

One of the most effective tools in determining your overall state of health is to measure your body's acid/alkaline balance. You can do so by purchasing pH strips or sticks and testing either your saliva or first morning urine. The pH scale goes from zero to 14, with zero being purely acid, 14 being purely alkaline, and 7 being "neutral" pH. Those with cancer, autoimmune diseases, or heavy-metal and chemical poisoning typically have an overall body pH below 7. In other words, their cells might not be getting enough oxygen, leading to an accumulation of toxins.

Fast food, processed food, preservatives, and chemicals such as MSG will always make us more acidic as well. We survive all the junk we eat because of the body's ability to rob the nutrients it needs—such as calcium, sodium, potassium, and magnesium—from other places such as soft tissues, organs, glands, bones, and teeth.

Research shows that diseases such as cancer are linked to an alkaline/acid balance. Thus, in order to resist disease, a balanced alkaline diet is key to our overall health.

Gifts from the Sea

When our bodies are in perfect alignment, we have the same exact balance of minerals as the sea. In *L'eau de mer, milieu organique* (which translates to *Seawater, Organic Medium*), René Quinton writes that it is only in the internal environment of our human system that we find the same mineral makeup and physiognomy as that of seawater. Our blood, lymphatic fluid, and plasma (the clear part of the blood) consists of 100 or more minerals and trace elements, the very same ones that circulate in the waves of the beautiful ocean.

The beneficial vitamins and minerals derived from the sea's gifts include vitamins A, B_1, B_2, and B_6; along with niacin, iodine, zinc, calcium, good sodium, potassium, and magnesium. Guess what that means? Seaweed is a great snack!

Imagine the potential that seaweed gives us in terms of replenishing all the minerals that are depleted due to cancer treatments. It's also known to contain specific molecules that slow cancer growth—as well as promote our natural killer (NK) cells, the important immune-system lymphocytes that help ward off disease and kill cancer cells.

I just love seaweed, and now that I've raised my kids on it, so do they. There are many different varieties for you to try:

- **Nori** are the seaweed sheets that are used in sushi restaurants to make the rolls. Nori is rich in long-chain omega-3 fatty acids, and is a potent inhibiter against inflammation.

- **Kombu** is often sold in a stick form that can be used in cooking. I use a kombu stick in all my grains and soups while they're simmering. The stick disburses minerals into the soup for more flavor and added health; when I'm done cooking, I simply remove it (it ends up looking like a piece of floppy seaweed that has washed up on a beach). Kombu releases all its fabulous vitamins and minerals into your food, and your kids never need to know a thing.

- **Wakame** promotes the death of cancer cells. This type of seaweed is brown when dried, but it turns soft and green when used in a broth for soup. This type of seaweed is added to miso soup, and it's very tasty.

- **Dulse** is a seasoning you can sprinkle on your soups, stews, and grains. It is slightly salty without being overpowering, and it offers a boost of minerals to your food. It's delicious and great for you.

- **Arame** and **hiziki** are my favorite varieties. They offer detoxification for your body, have been known to soften hard masses, benefit the thyroid, moisten dryness, promote healthy hair growth and soft skin, and actually prevent hair loss. A wonderful recipe using these types of seaweed is in my cookbook.

With all this talk of food you're probably unfamiliar with, I know it can be confusing when you're standing in the aisle of your grocery store. Therefore, I offer a comprehensive shopping list on my website that you can download and take with you.

Gaining a Sense of Yourself

When people ask me what I eat, my answer is simple: *I eat what makes me feel great.* I eat foods that promote life and health. I eat whole, natural foods in all their life-promoting, healing glory. As my guru Max used to say, "Eat it today, and if you feel good tomorrow, eat it again. If you feel bad tomorrow, don't eat it."

It's a simple mathematical equation: what we eat is how we feel. Yet it's amazing how many of us are unaware of what our bodies are telling us. We live so long with aches and pains that we accept them as "normal." I can't say this enough: *The body doesn't develop problems without good reason.* If you're having any kind of physical ailment, it's probably linked to what you're putting into your body, which would be food and beverages. This is, by the way, so easy to remedy. Don't make things so complicated and difficult. Screw the Twinkie. Haven't you already eaten all this crap before? You need another cheeseburger and fries like you need a hole in the head . . . or cancer.

One of my clients had the most horrific breath—the kind that's not from eating offensive-smelling foods. It was more like it had been caused by putrefaction or a rotten, leaky gut. I sent him for a scan, and sure enough, he had bile-duct cancer. It turns out that the duct was blocked by a tumor, forcing the bile up from his stomach to his mouth, where everyone could smell it. Breath tells me everything.

The body's warning system is a beautiful thing, so learn to be your own health detective. Be patient, though, as it does take some time. Look at the correlation between the signs and symptoms you're presented with and the food you eat. If you're downing pints of ice cream and/or drinking wine every night, and stimulating your already depleted adrenals with caffeine all day, it shouldn't shock you to discover that you're falling apart physically and emotionally—this would also explain why you need to be on all manner of prescriptions to prevent pain, suppress feelings, and get a good night's sleep.

Tune in to your body. Once you know what to look for, you'll recognize that it was probably trying to tell you something was wrong long before you went to the doctor's office.

With that being said, don't make yourself crazy as you obsess day and night over food (or anything, for that matter). One of my healers told me a story about two men, one of whom was walking down the beach whistling a tune, eating an ice-cream cone with a cherry on top; as the other one was sitting in a natural diner, digging through his macrobiotic meal and obsessively discarding fungus/yeast-causing mushrooms. Which guy lives longer? Answer: Sing a song . . . enjoy your new food. It is a privilege to feed your body this way, not a torture. If you do choose to eat an ice-cream cone one day, don't beat yourself up. Simply eat seaweed or kale the next day.

Now that you are starting to embrace the idea of transforming your eating habits and are learning to gain a new sense of yourself, it's time to focus on the environment in which you live every day.

CHAPTER SIX

"Recombobulate": Reinvent, Revamp, Refocus, and Renew

You've gotten through the hard part of eliminating low-energy, poor-quality food from your life. You've learned that the more you fill your beautiful body with vibrant, healing foods, the more you look and feel fantastic. Congratulations! Now it's time to keep the positive changes going.

I was walking through an airport one day when I saw a sign that said: RECOMBOBULATE. I just love this word. It brings to mind the way I find old furniture and clothing and revamp them in a creative way. Strangers often stop me and ask, "Where did you find that?" I'm excited to tell them that I only spent $10 or $20 on my outfit, but then I totally redesigned it. I think in some ways I do this with people, too.

Maybe you've been a bit *dis*combobulated since the diagnosis, or it's been even longer than that. If you've been feeling totally fragmented since all this began, it's high time for you to recombobulate.

Again, think of yourself as a garden, which you've been cultivating with love, patience, nurturing, and awareness. What does your garden need now: watering, seeding, or sodding? Above all, does it need weeding? Note that negative thought patterns in your life—such as anger, shame, inadequacy, insecurity, and simply not feeling good enough about yourself—rob you of vitality and healthy chi, just as weeds in a garden strangle the life force from precious fruits and vegetables. So if you need to clear this energy from your life, there's no time like the present to get to work. (Remember, I gave you all those great tips on emotional cleanses in Chapter 4.)

Do you know someone who instantly lights up a room the second he or she walks through the door? Well, you can be this way, too, regardless of what you've been through in the past. Take a look at me—although I've dealt with cancer for many years now, I've also been told that my energy is so positive that I'm able to share it with an entire room. Some might call this *joie de vivre* or charisma, but I call it positive chi or life-force energy. This energy can make an average-looking person much more attractive, it can lift the spirits of others, and it even has the power to heal. This mystery energy makes all things possible, and it is available to you right now.

You've been given the perfect opportunity to put yourself back together in an entirely new way. You can do so by reinventing, revamping, refocusing, and renewing. This chapter is full of fun tips that will help lead you to an exciting metamorphosis.

Unique as a Fingerprint

Before I talk about specific tips to recombobulate, I want to emphasize something: *We are so much more than doctors tell us we are.* It's important to believe that.

I always tell people that I don't buy into the bullshit of genes; we are all as unique as our fingerprints. I don't care what my ancestors had before me. I tell my doctors, "I am not your typical 'standard of care,' so don't treat me as such." I've never had the BRCA test done, which shows specific genetic mutations that are linked to increased cancer risk. I won't accept that or put it on my children. Instead, I tell them, "This isn't for you kids. You will never get cancer; your dad and I have taken it on for you. It isn't *about* you or *for* you."

I believe in mind over matter. I have a girlfriend whose always-positive attitude I love. She often says, "I'm not sure why, but I know I will never, ever get breast cancer." You know what? She won't. Just the words that come out of her mouth every day—*I will never get cancer*—seal her fate in concrete. She has no idea about her genes, nor does she care. Similarly, I have a knowing from deep inside that my kids will never get cancer. This is the seed I have planted for them.

Dr. David Servan-Schreiber doesn't buy into all the scientific bullying either. In his book *Anticancer,* he also recommends that we treat ourselves as unique individuals. He writes: "In short, the statistics we are shown on cancer survival don't distinguish between people who are satisfied with passively accepting the medical verdict and those who mobilize their own natural defenses."

I find it fascinating—and disturbing—that people who abuse their bodies are lumped together with individuals who have made enormous changes in their lives with diet, stress management, and emotional growth. This last group includes those of us who are kicking cancer's ass.

Re-create Your Look

Looking great translates to how you feel. Write this on your bathroom mirror right now: *I am beautiful.* And do whatever it takes to start believing it. (I wrote: *I am gorgeous; I am sexy; I am free to forgive;* and *I am safe, healed, and whole* on my own mirrors.)

I know you may feel like shit right now, and that some days you don't feel well enough to even leave the house. But when you do get that little bit of energy to go out, you *must* dress up and look great. You'll see what a difference it makes.

When you go for your treatments, go in looking smokin' hot, ready to take on the world. Don't you dare go in there with a look of defeat. No sweatpants! Studies have shown that how we dress affects our actual mood— so when you put on a pair of fabulous shoes, along with a pretty dress or a great suit (not to mention lingerie), you can't help but feel confident, sexy, strong, vital, and empowered.

I learned the importance of dressing for success from my husband during his cancer treatments. He totally changed his look from a conservative overweight man to a hip guy with cancer. The good news about Steve's weight loss during treatments was that later he was able to fit into a sleek black suit with a crisp white shirt and thin tie. He looked very sexy as he blasted his favorite hip-hop music in the car on the way to his treatments. Whether it was radiation or chemo, he appeared to be some cool-lookin' guy, going somewhere to kick ass (which is exactly what he was doing).

In your life before your diagnosis, you may have dressed like a slob, been overweight, or not really focused on your looks. That won't work now. Things need to change right this minute! So treat yourself: Go buy a new outfit. Create a new look. Throw out all those old, drab clothes. My motto is: "Less is more; buy quality, not quantity." If you lack funds, get creative and try secondhand stores—in fact, some of my favorite items are thrift-store revamps.

Don't let people see you looking sad, pathetic, or forlorn. "Poor thing . . . isn't it a shame?" is *not* what you want to hear them saying about you. You're not going to do very well if you have all those negative messages surrounding you. So instead, dress and carry yourself to elicit a positive response, such as: "Can you believe how great she looks? She doesn't even look sick!" or "What an incredibly strong person."

After leaving a room, I always want people to say, "Oh my God, she looks great." The positive energy behind these types of words strengthens us, even if we don't hear it directly. It's all about shifting the energy—and however you achieve this is up to you.

The opportunities for personal growth through this beautiful and imperative health-awakening journey are endless and tremendous. For example, even before you got diagnosed, you may have been feeling that you were in a rut. If that's the case, this is the perfect time to lift yourself up and create someone new and improved. There's no need to be submissive and weak. I learned to go against my nature, and you can, too. If you've always given up or been the victim, change it so that you're now an ass-kicker!

What the Bleep Do We Know!? is such a great movie because it shows that if you're the "victim," you'll attract more of that energy. If you're the "winner," though, so shall you win. Messages from movies and music can empower every cell in your body, so be sure to find the ones that inspire *you*, and draw strength from them when necessary.

Get in Kick-Ass Shape

In order to combat cancer, we must do all we can to keep our body, mind, and spirit performing optimally so that we can properly defend ourselves. To that end, I have immersed myself in alternative studies of the mind and body ever since my first diagnosis. This has proved to be an unbelievable asset to me. For example, I discovered that staying in peak condition through my surgeries and chemotherapies was much easier when I was in fighting shape physically.

Think of yourself like a prizefighter, a football player, or any serious athlete—your priority is to be in amazing shape so you can kick ass day after day. If you went into a fight or a game unprepared, would you expect to win or lose? How much abuse would you have to take before you decided to fight back?

For those of you who are a little overweight or not so fit, that doesn't matter. You can still get started now. Don't sit around wasting this health-awakening opportunity by feeling sorry for yourself or taking a backseat to the whole experience. Get up off the couch and do something proactive. Take up yoga, Pilates, or swimming. Or just walk with your dogs or a friend—this is a very therapeutic and grounding activity.

Breathing exercises are also very calming and good for strengthening the heart. The more oxygen our bodies have, the less chance there is for cancer to grow. The Art of Living Foundation is an organization that teaches breathing techniques, and it is in every state—just check online for classes offered in your area. The organization offers a four-day basic training course, which enables you to go once a week for free for the rest of your life. It's a great deal.

Trampoline jumping happens to be the number one exercise for lymphatic drainage; try dancing on a mini trampoline to fun music. Weights can prove to be too constricting, so make sure that if you use them (like I do), you use lighter ones or rubber bands, and then counteract the tightening of muscles with stretching or yoga. I suggest speed-walking over high-impact running, especially if you're going through surgeries or other therapies. Relatively gentle but steady exercise is best.

Chemotherapy may be damaging on the heart muscle, so you must strengthen it with breathing techniques and cardiovascular workouts. Many scientific studies have proven that cardio on the same day of chemo, when done before the treatment, can reduce the negative side effects of chemotherapy by as much as 50 percent.

I won't say, "You should consult with your physician here," since that somehow seems to be taken as, "You should ask your doctor's permission." Try checking in with your intuition first, and then discuss it with your physician, letting him know what you have in mind as an active participant in your healing process. If your doctor has any objections, hear him out, then use your newly gained sense to assess how you feel about his suggestions. There should be some room to compromise.

Earlier I told you about a darling older client of mine who had endured grueling chemotherapy regimens for five years. When her daughter called on me to work with her, I found all 90 pounds of this once-beautiful model bundled up on the sofa with a huge, swollen belly. She could barely move. I told her she must start pumping her lymphatic system, as all the fluid in her belly was stagnant lymph fluid. She said, "My doctor didn't tell me to exercise." I insisted she start with five minutes of walking every morning. It wasn't easy for her daughter to drag her out at first, but that five minutes led to three miles eventually. Between exercising, changing her food, and adding vitamin infusions, her quality of life changed dramatically.

If you're not sure where to start when it comes to exercise, again, I suggest that you just start walking. Or you could visit a YMCA or Cancer Wellness Center in your area, as they offer a variety of classes—many are inexpensive, and some are even free.

Cancer Wellness Centers offer group therapy as well. For me, though, I found it more effective to do my venting by physically working out instead of discussing how I was feeling with a group. It didn't boost my morale to hear accounts from others who were living or dying with cancer—I didn't want to be dragged down by defeatist stories, or by people staying stuck in their victim roles or complaining. Your experience may be different, however; perhaps you'll want to join a group in the beginning or all the way through your journey. It's up to you.

Be careful when listening to others. To this day, for instance, I tell doctors and nurses not to go down the long list of side effects I could or should be having from treatments. I say, "I'll tell you, don't tell me." I've had minimal side effects over the years, and I want to keep it that way. I feel it's best not to put the intention in our heads—we must be the creator of our own movies.

Revamp Your Car

While you're getting your body into kick-ass shape, you must clean up your surrounding environment as well. My mother used to say, "Our automobiles represent our emotional bodies." I believe this to be true. Many times I have stressed-out clients come to me complaining that their lives are falling apart. Sure enough, when I look at their cars, they seem to somehow match how my clients feel. So if you have a vehicle that continues to attract accidents, keeps breaking down, or is generally a big mess, this could be a sign to clean up your life and slow down.

I've had dreams in the past where I'm speeding downhill and the brakes won't work . . . I can't slow down. I am actually frightened in these dreams, and it feels like a terrifying roller-coaster ride. I know when I wake up that I've been given a message: I need to slow down in my life or something bad will happen.

We should always listen to our dreams. I didn't listen to a "slow down" dream once, and I hit a woman on a bike. (She wasn't hurt, thank God.) The dream immediately came to mind, and I realized that my car, being a representation of my emotional body, was totally out of control. Like so many of us, I was rushing through life with no time to enjoy the precious moment. I was being told that I must slow down, breathe, and take time to notice the beauty around me.

Here's an interesting side note: After the surgery to remove my brain tumor, I came out to a car that had been hit from behind while parked in the hospital lot—and when I got home, my computer had totally crashed. I had to laugh at the symbolism of it all. So clean up your car, throw away all the clutter, take it in for a tune-up, and detail it if you can. It is very therapeutic to wash and clean your car. Listen to your body, car, and even computer, as they speak to you and act as extensions of your self.

Renew Your Home

According to the art of *feng shui,* our homes reflect our physical and emotional states. This concept proved true for me when I was diagnosed with bone and lung cancer. Our basement had flooded a year earlier, and we hadn't gotten around to fixing it up yet. Upon being diagnosed, one of my natural doctors told me it was imperative to get that basement cleaned up immediately because it represented the foundation of my life. I already knew this from the way I was feeling . . . so uprooted, ungrounded, disorganized, and discombobulated. The minute the basement was finished, I felt so much better. It was no coincidence that this project was completed at the same time as my last round of chemo.

In the end, that basement flooding, which seemed like a catastrophe at the time, ended up being a blessing in disguise. I cleaned out so much unnecessary junk that I was inspired to go through the entire house, clearing out all the excess clutter that was dragging me down. From the junk drawers in the kitchen, to nightstands littered with magazines in the master bedroom, it was time to eliminate the sky-high piles in my life.

I had a client once who called me after having just been diagnosed with lymphoma. Although she was understandably upset, I told her that she was actually lucky and should take this as the health-awakening opportunity that it was. I went to her home to clear out all the inflammation-causing foods, as they are the number one issue with lymphoma. (It's no surprise we are seeing lymphoma pop up so much more these days in our "inflammation nation.") I saw that not only was she wrapped in too much fat on her physical body, but her home was also wrapped in excess material things as well.

I quickly went to work on this woman's body and her home. She and I worked together, which is very empowering for my clients. Due to her desperate diagnosis, she was a willing and more-than-able participant; we ended up throwing out 22 industrial garbage bags of unnecessary stuff from her kitchen, living room, and family room. She was in remission in six weeks with absolutely no treatments. As an added bonus, she lost about 20 pounds.

My advice: Give your home a thorough cleaning, devoting an entire weekend to the process. (Don't overwhelm yourself, though—start with one room at a time.) Get rid of excess papers, clothes, and books; along with unused furniture from your basement, attic, or garage. A good rule of thumb is that anything you haven't used or worn in the last year goes to Goodwill.

Remember, gluttony is one of the seven deadly sins. Don't sit around and wallow in the muck, and don't live in a sick house. *Let go.* You will feel lighter, and your body will respond positively to the energy of a clear, clutter-free home and environment.

Reinvent Your Spirit

Many of us, especially women, make choices in early adulthood to get married and raise a family, or to enter into the workforce—and we give up pieces of ourselves along the way. This is also true for men who may have gone to work in their father's business or had to meet the high expectations of parents. Consequently, lots of us have never been able to fully realize our own dreams.

Now is the time to clean out your spirit by bringing to light your long-ago buried desires. You may have wanted to become an artist, musician, photographer, or even a magician at one time. As crazy as it may seem, it's time to take your dreams out and dust them off, whatever they may be. What is your secret fantasy? Get giddy like a child just thinking about the peace you'll feel when you fulfill it now.

Cancer gives you the gift of freedom from the old constraints that bound you. What if you die? What legacy would you leave? Throw all caution to the wind. Of the many clients I've consulted with cancer, rarely have I come across any who have followed their hearts' desires thus far. One of them was actually embarrassed to tell me that he had wanted to play the saxophone when he was younger. I encouraged him to take lessons, and he did start playing. He's now in a part-time band and having a ball.

One of my own dreams was to be onstage, empowering a whole audience of people on a health-awakening journey like me. I also dreamed of writing inspirational books and plays. The problem was that I had a long laundry list of fears to fail by, so I easily gave up my dreams. I hid them away.

Since I first found Louise Hay's little blue book years ago, I not only dreamed of meeting her, but of being published by her company as well. I'll never forget the day I decided to go for it. My fears were doing their best to stop me, until I screamed at them to "Stop!" If fears could be shocked, they were. I then marched into my home and contacted Hay House. In my proposal, I let them know that they were the only publisher for me. Now that my book has been published, it proves that all my old excuses only served to delay my dream from coming true. Excuses are an illusion; dreams are reality.

If you have a vision in your head that just won't go away, you must pay attention to it. Go after your dream today. I truly feel like cancer kept hitting me over the head until I got it. Getting diagnosed with a disease that threatened my whole existence certainly forced me to take a good look at myself and see what was truly important. I'm still reaching for more of my dreams—when I get side-tracked, I remind myself that I will fulfill my destiny as God intended in this lifetime, and so shall you.

For those of you going through a health-awakening experience right now, my advice is to be open to developing a new side of yourself. Some of you may feel as if you're being ripped open, while others will welcome growth and change easily. I was never one who liked growing pains; perhaps this is why the universe gave me so many of them, so I could learn to enjoy them.

Whenever my kids complain that things are too tough between school, jobs, and sports, I tell them that there is nothing else they need to do and nowhere else they need to be. There is only this moment, and in it we find the real "work." In other words, we all have our individual mountains of mud to deal with, and we can either complain about the mess or have fun like a child and make mud pies. The process can take our entire lifetime or many lifetimes, so we might as well enjoy the ride.

I once heard singer John Mayer say, "In life, people trip. Most people fall, but some people turn that trip into a beautiful dance." And when you fall out of a pose in yoga, they say, "Fall with grace." So fall into something new and wonderful with grace.

Travel to a place you've always dreamed of seeing, enroll in a class you've always wanted to take, learn about something that excites and intrigues you. I recently went dirt-bike riding, for instance, and it was so much fun to triumph over something new and scary. I fell more than a few times, but it felt so liberating. When I realized it couldn't kill me to fall on the soft dirt or grass, I let go and laughed till I cried. I found that the harder I gripped the handles of the bike, the more it would throw me off. This is similar to a horse (or even life itself)—when it senses your fear as you hold on too tightly, you restrict the flow and natural process of a beautiful ride. Next on my thrill list is learning to "drop in" on a skateboard. I'll have to cushion myself like the Michelin Man, but I will conquer.

The good news is that you can now focus on your purpose rather than your problems. You get to live as though you never know when you will leave this earth, and turn the fear of dying into the exhilaration of living.

Refocus the Warrior

The world of cancer can be such a lonely one. For the most part, we're on this path all alone. I had my husband right there to hold me and talk me through it, but still, the silence was deafening. It was still only me who was actually going through it, me who needed to muster up the strength and power to fight every day.

I use the word *fight*, but it's really about *balance*. In yin and yang, you find the balance between the male and female sides of everything that exists. In yoga, there is something called *sukha* (ease, joy, or sweetness) and *sthira* (steady, firm, or sour). This is a balance between the effort or the more difficult part of the pose, and the ease or the sweet part of the pose.

The fight against cancer is like taking a walk on a tightrope. You must learn the art of surrendering your grip with elegance and grace as you call on your focus, brute strength, and fortitude. It takes equal parts of all these energies if you are to survive. It's much like the ancient Chinese art of qigong, in which great masters teach never to fight in anger, but rather to flow like water through your enemy. Like a dance, you gently move with your attacker, not against him.

It's time to call on the warrior. After all, it takes courage, conviction, and plenty of guts to battle cancer. It's a really ballsy move to look that disease in the eye and say, "I'm gonna kick your ass." Gather all your weapons—your arsenal of traditional treatments combined with natural remedies, protocols, foods, and alternative healers. Lock, load, and dance!

In addition, it helps to find movies that inspire and uplift your spirit. Give these a try: *Crouching Tiger, Hidden Dragon; Peaceful Warrior; Cinderella Man;* and even *Rocky,* as funny as it sounds. Personally, I liked *Lara Croft: Tomb Raider* with Angelina Jolie for a jolt of kick-ass adrenaline.

Speaking of movies, a really great one to watch is National Geographic's *Amazing Planet: Destructive Forces.* As I watched this documentary, I was amazed by how I could compare what happened in nature to what I was going through. You see, catastrophe has been the creator of the most beautiful, mesmerizing, and astounding things throughout history. You only need to look at the Grand Canyon to know that this is true. Out of horrific disasters come the most breathtaking results, such as rivers, valleys, and mountain ranges.

All cycles of destruction and upheaval create miraculous examples of peace, calm, and beauty. This is the Cycle of Life: birth, life, destruction, death, and then rebirth. This doesn't necessarily mean a physical death of the human body; it may just be a death of a piece of you that you have simply outgrown. Think of it like a snake shedding its old skin.

Look to nature to balance your warrior sides in your new world.

Rewrite the Messages to Yourself

Some of the emotional characteristics associated with cancer are feelings of loneliness, fear of expressing emotions, guilt, or low self-esteem. Most of us have a negative radio station that plays over and over. We must change the station; our lives depend upon it.

So many of us get so comfortable in our own shit that we don't want to let it go, in more ways than one. We come up with every excuse as to why we cannot work through it. We believe our stories, which are composed of nothing more than old thoughts, and we let them develop into negative manifestations in the body.

I recently saw a client who was so negative . . . everything I suggested to her was "impossible." Have you ever met someone like this? She was full of excuses as to why things could not be done. I finally told her, "Well, then, looks like you're enjoying the pain." She looked at me in shock. I then suggested that she watch *The Secret* in her home all day and night just to start the positive-energy ball rolling.

We are the most powerful force on the planet—we can create whatever we need. Our thoughts are creative, our words are more creative, and our actions are the most creative. So think healthy; speak healthy; write healthy; and, above all, act healthy. Once my client started to see life as a blessing, her entire reality shifted. She left that day in tears at all the work that lay ahead for her, but she did it. And that once-negative woman is now teaching health and healing to others.

I created a necklace for myself that says I AM on the top, and on the back (the side that touches my chest) is inscribed PERFECT HEALTH. I also gave myself powerful little "love notes," which helped me in so many ways. I taped them all over the house and wrote them on mirrors with lipstick. I even wrote them on the bags of chemotherapy meds as they dripped in to my veins.

Find positive sayings to surround yourself with; say them every day in any way, sing them, shout them, think them, and read them repeatedly. Do whatever it takes to reclaim your power and change your mind. Try using the following, which are some of my all-time favorite quotes (you can also make up your own):

"Look well into thyself;
there is a source of strength which will always spring up
if thou wilt always look there."

— MARCUS AURELIUS

"I am the master of my fate: I am the captain of my soul."

— FROM "INVICTUS," BY WILLIAM ERNEST HENLEY
(NELSON MANDELA SAID THAT THIS POEM, AND THESE
LINES IN PARTICULAR, SUSTAINED HIM IN PRISON)

"I am free of all limits; God I am, love I am, perfect health I am."

— The I AM Temple

"I lovingly forgive and release all of the past. I choose to fill my world with joy. I love and approve of myself."

— from Heal Your Body, by Louise L. Hay

Stay on Your Own Mat

"Stay on your own mat" is a saying I learned in yoga. Boy, have I needed it! Sometimes my practice is great, while other times it's like that of a child. And I have to start all over again every time I have a surgery—similar to Humpty Dumpty, I must put myself back together again. I could never measure myself by looking at other yogis in the room, or I would be so frustrated that I'd never go to class.

The day I wrote this segment of the book, I was of course put to the test. I went to a very challenging class with one of my favorite teachers, who is tough as nails. In walked a beautiful friend of mine from my yoga-teacher training, and she placed her mat directly in front of me. I was prepared to stay on my own mat; and, as always, deviate my practice from that of the teacher and other students, making it suitable for what I was feeling that particular day. But I started to watch my friend a little too much, and I fell off my mat literally and figuratively. I was admiring her gorgeous flow and balance, so I inevitably started tripping all over myself. I actually laughed out loud as I realized what was happening. Just when we become complacent or cocky on our path, we're forced to put down our egos and look at ourselves on an even deeper level.

It's the same with cancer: I never wanted to know about the how, when, where, and why of anyone else's cancer situation. As I've said before, I believe that everyone is as unique as his or her fingerprint. Thus, there is not any one way of life that suits everyone. No one has the exact same type of cancer as you . . . they don't have the same emotional issues . . . they don't have the same past or mother and father. Their holding patterns are totally different from yours. The natural doctor who helped me may not be good for you, the yoga that helped your neighbor through her breast cancer may not be great for you. What resonates with *you?*

Truly honor thyself and stay on your own mat . . . and get ready to turn yourself inside out in your own very unique way!

CHAPTER SEVEN

Turning Yourself Inside Out

You should be noticing positive changes in many areas of your life, particularly since you've learned how to reinvent and refocus yourself personally as well as renew and revamp your physical surroundings. As you shed some of the old and continue to grow, you'll be ever expanding in exciting new directions.

Turning ourselves inside out is a must. In fact, it's an inevitable process when we're faced with something as motivating as cancer. It inevitably took me a long time to see that my healing depended on digging in deep at a root level. Just like a plumber who can't fix a sink until he gets the greasy hairy blob out of the way, I ultimately had no choice but to work on repairing the damage that had been done to me for so many years. I don't know why I couldn't get it sooner—I just kept getting beaten over the head with the same message through each diagnosis.

I ultimately learned that it's extremely important to do the following:

- Admit that there is something wrong on an emotional level.

- Be willing to dig in and do the real work.

- Realize that what you dislike in others you typically find and dislike in yourself.

- Use events that upset you as an opportunity for growth.

- Forgive anyone who has hurt you. This doesn't mean that you necessarily need to engage in a relationship with them, but you do need to *truly* forgive them.

- Stop the blame game.

- Accept things and people you cannot change, and know you can only change yourself.

- Heal emotionally as well as physically at all costs, even if that means disconnecting from certain individuals.

- Connect with your source, the light, or your higher power through prayer and meditation. Remember to let go and let God, and that you are never alone.

Sounds easy, right? You might even be sarcastically asking, "Is that all?"

No, that's *not* all. You're going to have to create your own list of emotional challenges, and then do whatever is necessary to overcome them, one step at a time. Whether it's anger, obsessive-compulsive disorder, control issues, depression, envy, or the always-crushing victim trap, you must find a way to take this health-awakening opportunity to turn yourself inside out and save your life. As I've said many times throughout this book, you are lucky. You *get* to do this. Yay, you!

The Codependency Connection

When you're diagnosed with a major disease like cancer, you can bet that it's typically related to some emotional junk from the past. You can stay in denial if you like, but eventually you're going to have to look at it.

I know what I'm speaking of here. When I was just a teenager, I changed my way of life to a healthier one outwardly; but inside, my emotional baggage was killing me. I couldn't understand why I was consistently in abusive relationships that drained me of everything I had.

I come from a long line of addictive family members, and I've also had a lot of friendships and intimate relationships with addicts. I was thrilled to find a great book, *Codependent No More* by Melody Beattie. Wow, I had never seen anything that described me so perfectly. I also found codependency meetings to be extremely helpful. It was such a relief to know that there were others like me, I wasn't crazy, and help was available.

I eventually stopped going to the meetings when I needed them most. I moved to Chicago to live and work with my brother . . . who was, of course, an addict.

Today when I meet with clients with breast cancer, I quite often see the common codependency thread—the women who come to me are typically drained in the same way that I once was. The signs and symptoms are all too familiar:

- Continually seeking approval or affirmations from others

- A lack of self-confidence in making decisions, and no sense of power in making choices

- Feelings of fear, guilt, inadequacy, hurt, and shame that are invalidated

- Dependency on others and fear of abandonment

- Confusion between love and pity

- The tendency to look for victims to help

- Rigidity and the need to control

- A tendency to take on the victim role

- A feeling of responsibility for other people's feelings and needs

- The loss of interest in one's own life when involved in someone else's

- The need to stay in abusive relationships that don't work in order to keep others' "love"

Typically, we women seem to fit these patterns much more than men do, since we're raised to be little caretakers.

One thing is for sure: you don't become ill without having "dis-ease," which is a term Louise Hay often uses. In her book *Heal Your Body,* Louise connects the emotional component of cancer to deep hurt and long-standing resentment, secrets, or grief. I'd also venture to say that most women who get a diagnosis of breast cancer would greatly benefit by reading about, or working with, some form of codependency counseling. However, the innate desire to overnurture is not exclusive to people with breast cancer—many different types of diagnoses seem to have this common thread.

It's no surprise that most of my relationships were with addicts. I grew up in an emotionally abusive home, never feeling the love and acceptance a child so desperately needs, which contributed to a crack in my emotional core. Because I was predisposed to trauma and the feeling of constant heartbreak from a very young age, I continued to attract more of what I was familiar with. As an adult, when societal pressures, relationship issues, everyday stress, and emotional wounds arose, I was overly sensitive and unequipped to process them in a healthy way. I've heard this referred to as the "C personality" (the C stands for "cancer").

When I was originally diagnosed, many old feelings from a lifetime of trauma emerged. I must have been holding on to them for a rainy day. I was overwhelmed at first; then I took a look at the giant mountain of emotional garbage in front of me, pulled on my waders, and started digging into the muck.

Even now, just when I think I've climbed up and out of the garbage dump—and taken a bath to wash myself clean of all the dirt—oops, there I go again, back down in it. Time for more slipping and sliding around in deeply rooted emotional pain from the past. But I find patience and compassion in knowing that the deep emotional work is necessary in order for me to survive, thrive, and continue to grow.

Your Body Speaks

Your body speaks to you through physical, emotional, and energetic manifestations . . . are you listening? The experience is different for everyone, but your body will absolutely tell you, in a language only you can understand, exactly what is wrong and what it needs. You will have to assess the physical and emotional work that's necessary for *you*.

For me, this is no game; it is a matter of life and death. After all these years, I know how my body works, and that an emotional trauma is more detrimental than eating a burger and fries could ever be (and you know from Chapter 5 how I feel about that kind of food). Personally, holding on to old hurt and pain is like taking a match to kerosene. Poof, it causes cancer.

Before I was ever diagnosed, my body told me that there was a problem on a physical level. I had an unbearable pain in my back—it felt as if a dagger was constantly stabbing straight through me, from front to back. I had strange bumps all over my shoulders that had formed as my body's way of expressing toxins. I also started hacking up mucus like a six-foot-tall man who smokes . . . not so attractive.

I decided to look to my questionable past for the answers. Growing up, I ate a typical American diet of Twinkies, macaroni and cheese, and Jack in the Box (shh, don't tell). The excessive amounts of sugars, preservatives, antibiotics, steroids, and other chemicals in my mostly processed diet had created a deficit in my health. As you know, I believe that what we put in, we get out. In this case, what I was putting in, I *wasn't* getting out: I developed persistent constipation. Physical stress hindered my body to the point that my organs and lymphatic system had become sluggish and unable to efficiently cleanse, thereby contributing to a buildup of toxins. What resulted from this combination was chronic inflammation.

Inflammation is a complicated biochemical process that happens at the cellular level, which in turn compromises your cells' ability to regenerate and heal. It can be caused by your diet, lifestyle, emotions, and even relationship history. This hot topic is popping up everywhere, and is linked to all sorts of diseases, such as diabetes, arthritis, fibromyalgia, migraines, asthma, and—you got it—cancer.

Of course, food was only a part of the equation. As I've already discussed in this book, there is always an emotional manifestation connected with disease. So the emotionally wounded state I grew up in, along with the physical stress from years of a poor-quality diet, was the recipe for a Molotov cocktail of sorts that caused cancer.

Chinese medicine teaches that each organ is energetically linked to an emotion. For instance:

- large intestine/lungs = grief/sadness
- kidney/bladder = fear/anxiety
- spleen/stomach = worry
- liver/gallbladder = anger/frustration
- small intestine/heart = joy/shock

On an energetic level, I was experiencing pain on the right side of my body because it is the masculine and giving side. The left side is the feminine, receiving side. I was giving much more than I was receiving, and I was angry about it to boot.

Anger, frustration, and resentment had really taken its toll on me over the years. This led to a constriction of energy flow on my right side, creating congestion in my liver, located just below the breast. The stagnant, angry energy was actually backing up from the liver into my breast, and I could feel it. So the emotional issues led to energetic issues, which in essence caused a physical problem. Now can you begin to understand how that works?

It's just like the childhood song that tells us about the ankle bone being connected to the shinbone, and the shinbone being connected to the knee bone . . . every part of us is connected and interconnected. Each organ affects the other; and our emotions, energy, and physical selves must all be in balance to work harmoniously. If one component is off-kilter, the rest will quickly suffer.

It can be frustrating to work on energetic and emotional levels. It's sort of like playing *Monopoly*—just when you think you've made it all the way around the board and can't wait to collect $200, you roll the dice and land on "Go to Jail." Oh shit, you have to go all the way back, start over, and do it again. You don't even get the $200. You've been caught, snagged, and triggered by old anger, trauma, or grief. Just when you think you're safe, you're pulled back into a mountain of muck. This typically happens around the holidays . . . that's why they were created, right? Holidays are an advanced course in emotional acceptance and surrender—don't you just love 'em?

I recommend that you take the time to analyze where you are right now. Honestly look at all physical or emotional manifestations, as well as energy blocks you might have in your body. Then look at your lifestyle choices, along with what you're consuming on a daily basis. Take an inventory of all the prescription medications you're on, including sleep aids, suppressants, anxiety pills, and pain medications (this is sure to be an eye-opening experience).

Remember the equation we've been talking about? What you put in—in terms of food, medications, emotions, and energy—is truly what you'll get out. It's not a guessing game; you will be the first to know when your body is out of balance because it will throw a kicking-and-screaming temper tantrum.

When we ignore the signs our bodies so generously give us, we inevitably wind up with a much bigger prob lem than we started with. The pain then leads us to search for answers. Keep in mind that your answers will be different from mine, and will reveal themselves to you in your own unique ways.

The Inside-Out Method

While Elisabeth Kübler-Ross famously identified the five stages of grief, I have my own version of the Grief Cycle. I call it the "Inside-Out Method." This is what I've personally experienced through the process of turning myself inside out:

— It begins with *fear.* Fear is a distressing emotion aroused by impending danger, evil, or pain; the fear of the unknown is a gripping emotion as it gets you in its clutches and refuses to let go. The word *panic* can be traced back to *Panikos,* meaning "of Pan," the Greek god who sometimes caused intense, sudden, and mindless fear. Anyone who has had a diagnosis of cancer can relate to this. The good news is that *fear* also stands for "fiction experienced as reality." Ha ha, you must laugh at fear, as it's all an illusion of things that most often never come to pass. Unfortunately, most of our worst decisions are made in the moment of fear.

Fear was a great trigger from my old childhood traumas. When I was first diagnosed, even though I was a grown woman, I became physically ill at the thought of being left alone. My old childhood trauma reemerged in the face of the cancer trauma. I found comfort in creating "Mother Love," by imagining Mother Earth protecting me so that I need never feel alone: I would plant my belly in the grass and picture my umbilical cord growing like a tree root into the universal mother. I'd lie there breathing as the earth cradled and calmed me. As it embraced me, I felt safe.

— Then comes the *shock*. Shock is a sudden or violent disturbance of the mind, emotions, or sensibilities. Shock is traumatic because it can leave long-lasting scars with far-reaching effects on a cellular level. This is an emotion I'm used to—and when I experienced the shock of being diagnosed, all that old shock/trauma I'd experienced as a child came flooding back.

— Soon to follow is *denial*. Denial is the refusal to recognize or acknowledge. It's a disbelief in the existence or reality of something. I became an expert in the denial game: no matter how much abuse I took growing up, I would always go back for more, kind of like a loyal dog. And when I was first diagnosed, it was so tough to accept that this was happening to me.

— Rearing its ugly head next comes *anger,* which the dictionary defines as "a strong feeling of displeasure and belligerence aroused by being wronged." This emotion was no stranger to me. I was in a playwriting workshop when the teacher wrote on the board, *I Am Born in . . . .* and asked us to finish the statement in a play form. I didn't even give it a second thought—my title was *I Was Born in Anger.* All that old anger energy emerged for me while I dealt with cold, uncaring, and sometimes even abusive doctors throughout my diagnosis. Most of all, I was so angry to know deep in my soul that anger had contributed to cancer.

I am in no way saying that if you are dealing with emotional or physical stress, or grew up in a traumatic way, then you're automatically a candidate for cancer. My advice is to use anger for its motivational energy—but then work through it, bless it, and move on.

— *Surrender/acceptance* means to give yourself up to some influence, course, or emotion; to let go fully without attachment to the outcome. It's the most challenging work, as it requires patience and persistence and self-love. This is the stage I aspire to be at, and it's a work in progress. To be able to let go with love is such a beautiful concept, but I'd be lying if I said that I've mastered it. (I talk more about surrender in the next section.)

The Inside-Out Method is not an easy or short process, but don't let that stop you. Don't stay stuck—purge it, baby! Look your mountain of muck straight in the eye, and warn it that you are ready to dig as deep as it takes, and for as long as it takes, until you are as clear and healthy as you can be. Remember, this is your life's work, so have fun and enjoy the moment.

Time to Surrender

Surrendering is the perfect recipe for contentment. Why, then, is this task of letting go and moving on so much easier for some than it is for others?

It wasn't until my third go-round with cancer that I truly understood why I'd attracted it into my life. One day while meditating, I received the vision of a key. I went to my natural doctor to help interpret what this could mean, and we both felt that I was ready to open Pandora's box, if that's what it took, in order to find the answers to the recurring cancer in my life.

The following day I went into my special space to do some yoga and look for some more clues. As I was digging through some old CDs to play, I saw one by Caroline Myss called *Personal Healing*. I remembered going to her workshop with Dr. Wayne Dyer when I had first been diagnosed four years earlier, but I didn't remember buying this CD at all. I pressed Play.

The program began with a dedication to a woman named Penny who had died of breast cancer. I was just about to jump up and turn it off—the last thing I needed to hear was another story about cancer, especially if the person was dead. Yet something wouldn't let me move off my mat, so I stayed put and listened. I'm so glad I did, since it was by far the most valuable information I received through my healing transformation.

First Caroline spoke of some people's need to stay sick because, unconsciously, they might be getting something out of it. I saw how I might have been doing this so I could get the love I so desperately wanted from my family. I thought, *I won't do that anymore.*

Then she started to talk about the alchemy we do for ourselves. This sounded just like me, the queen of natural doctors, healing, tinctures, herbs, and remedies. My ears perked up when she said, "You can go to the ends of the earth for the most potent form of herb, tincture, or essential oil." I was anxiously waiting to hear where I needed to go next for the most miraculous potion on the face of the planet, when she said, "It's forgiveness. The remedy is simple: if you don't get rid of your bitter heart and forgive, nothing will work."

I immediately stood up and said out loud, "Okay, I'll do it. I will forgive. If that's what it takes, I can do that. If Caroline says to do it, I will." I was gung ho and ready to call the person I most needed to forgive: my mother.

Then the voice on the CD warned about the struggle between the ego and the spirit. Isn't that funny? This is exactly what was happening—my ego was taking out all the old pictures to show my spirit. My ego reminded my spirit, "You know what your mother will say. She will say what she said last time you tried to forgive her: 'I forgive you too, Dena,' in that patronizing way of hers. Remember the egotistical and accusatory way she said it? Yep, she will do it again."

But my spirit did exactly what Caroline said it would. "I don't care," it responded. "I must forgive her. My life depends upon it." I decided to make the call—but before I did, I sent my mother Caroline's CD, in the hopes that she would listen to it and better understand where I was coming from, and not hurt me as my ego feared she would. No such luck. When I told her, "Mom, I forgive you," she replied, "I forgive you, too," just like my ego warned. I now understand that she couldn't help herself . . . she was in *her* ego.

After the frustrating call, I went upstairs to my bathroom to blow-dry my hair, and I started to yell at God. "You think it's funny?!" I screamed. Then, through my tears, I laughed at the hypocrisy of it all. "It's all so cleverly done," I heard myself say. "So many twists and turns in dark alleys. I have the worst mother on the planet, I get cancer, and the only way to heal myself is through her.

What could You possibly have been thinking when You designed my life's plan?"

At this point, my husband walked in. He said, "Dena, I think you're confusing forgiveness with relationship." It was as if someone had turned on the proverbial lightbulb. All at once, the room went from dark to bright. *I got it.* God couldn't have possibly meant that I needed to stay in an unhealthy and dysfunctional relationship. I could forgive my mother and even love her, but not be in a relationship with her. This would take work—the addiction to the dysfunction was strong, and I knew it wasn't going to be easy for me to break free from this emotional web. Surrendering would be a process, but I was determined to accomplish this surrendering business in this lifetime.

●○●

I have also experienced physical surrender. What I mean by that is that I've had healers work on me at such an intense level that I've actually felt a strong unblocking of energy from past trauma leave my body. I call this process "unwinding the story" or "peeling the onion." It's frightening at times, and this process takes courage. I compare it to riding a bull; it's challenging both physically and emotionally, but in the end it's worth every painful tear shed.

My brother, who chose to surrender to drugs instead of doing any physical and emotional work, used to say, "Why would I want to dig up all that shit now? Let's get high instead." My reply was, "I'd rather deal with it now. In no way do I want to come back to look at these same lessons again."

It is in surrendering that change and growth are possible. I made a choice in this lifetime to learn the lessons of letting go. Although I work to release my pain, fear, and worries—and focus more on the present with love, joy, and health—I'd be lying if I said I didn't still have drama.

It's true, we wouldn't watch a movie without the drama. Any film that's all love and joy, completely devoid of conflict, is boring. We should keep that in mind when dealing with our own personal challenges. We can work on not getting overly involved, reminding ourselves that it's just part of the plot of our own life movie.

Julia Cameron profoundly writes about the power of surrender in her beautiful book *Transitions: Prayers and Declarations for a Changing Life* (Tarcher/Putnam, 1999):

The one change we cannot change is change itself. No moment, however perfect, can be maintained. Life moves on and moves us with it. We are all works in progress, all developing parts of a perfect plan. Only as we surrender to change can we find permanence and peace. Only by being open to the fierce flow of life can we find the steadying current. The one thing that remains the same is that nothing remains the same. As we accept and acknowledge life's passing nature, we are freed to cherish the moments that pass in bittersweet glory. No matter how difficult, life is beautiful. No matter how beautiful, life is difficult. This is the great paradox that opens the heart and brings compassion. We are all travelers on the vast and shifting sands of time. We are inconsequential and important, very small and very large. Our transitions are like octaves building brilliantly upon each other. We are life's music, so let us dance.

Be Selfish

I like to share the following story with many of my clients, especially those with cancer: A woman's husband had been killed at war, so she was forced to take care of herself and their five children on her own. She tried to stay strong and worked very hard just to survive. One day she came back to her children after a long day looking for work with one fragile egg in her hand.

The children cried with joy when they saw the beautiful egg. They watched their mother crack it open ever so carefully, cook it up, and eat the whole thing herself. They started to cry and asked her, "How could you do that? We're starving."

She simply replied, "If I don't have enough strength to survive, you will all perish."

Each cancer has its own lessons. In terms of breast cancer, the breast is the mothering aspect of our physical bodies and is by nature giving and nurturing. It is no wonder that so many women with breast cancer are depleted from giving, caring, sharing, making, and fixing everything and everyone around them.

Through this health-awakening process, I hope you've discovered that *you are all there is.* You are the most important person in your life; it would cost a fortune to replace you. In my particular situation, my house would need a full-time cook, babysitter, housekeeper, driver, friend, advisor/psychologist, and doctor/healer. We are all being pulled in a million different directions, be it at work or at home, and this can be very draining.

Reclaiming the ability to live for you might be difficult at first, even if you're single and don't have children. There are still people depending on you every day, right? Well, tell them to get lost. For the first time in 15 years, I had to put my husband and kids *after* me. Then if I had enough time and energy to spare after being with my immediate family, I could share myself with friends or clients. I've come to take this part of my healing very seriously, and I hope you will, too.

Make sure you take time for *you:* sleep when you're tired, eat when you're hungry, play when you feel lighthearted, and cry when you need to mourn. Find the freedom to develop a new way of life that revolves around *you* as much as you can.

Speaking of sleep, I learned a fascinating tidbit at The Raj health spa in Iowa, where I was fortunate enough to spend four glorious days immersed in Ayurvedic traditions—including transcendental meditation, the detoxifying treatments of *Panchakarma*, and delicious vegetarian healing fare. Ayurveda believes in three *doshas* called *pitta, vata,* and *kapha.* Kapha is described as the heavy or inactive hours, a time that is great for winding down or resting. The kapha hour is from 6 to 10 P.M., so it's best to eat your dinner before 6 and then take an after-dinner stroll as you wind down for the evening. The idea is to be in bed by 9:30, with lights out at 10:00. This ensures that you get the benefit of all eight hours of healing sleep your body so desperately needs.

When people tell me that they're on sleeping pills, I ask, "What time do you go to bed?" Typically, the answer is midnight or 1 A.M. Well, there's no way to get a good night's sleep when we're up past kapha hour. After kapha hour comes vata hour, which is all about high energy. In essence, when we stay up past 10 P.M., our bodies get reenergized, thereby making sleep impossible. At midnight, it becomes pitta hour, which is "fire in the belly." This is why we find ourselves sneaking downstairs for a midnight snack.

If your goal is to eliminate the pill popping and receive the maximum healing energy for your organs throughout the night, then do yourself a favor and go to bed at 10. Sweet dreams. . . .

Learn to Say No and Speak Your Truth

My very dear friend and business partner taught me a sentence that has proved to be very useful for creating healthy boundaries in my life. Here it is: "No, that's not going to work for me." I loved this so much that I wrote it down and taped it to every phone in my house.

Women in general have a difficult time saying no, as our society has raised us to be "nice," and saying no isn't "nice." (Of course, men can have a hard time saying no, too.) Nevertheless, even our families and our perfect little children need to hear us say it—we should practice saying it in the mirror if we have to.

I will warn you now that no one likes it when you start to change from a yes-girl to a no-girl. I will also tell you that this small two-letter word is imperative for your health if you're going to change the old patterns that hold you hostage. Each time you invalidate yourself and say yes when you want to say no, you're only adding to unhealthy emotional energy such as anger, frustration, resentment, and grief. Remember, this stuck energy affects you on a cellular level.

Change can be scary—you may feel like I did: *If I don't help, fix, and save others, will they still love me?* The first step is to become aware of these feelings. Don't stuff them. Acknowledge that they exist. If your body starts to scream at you with physical pain, you know it has manifested from some stress in your life. You might have symptoms such as difficulty taking a full deep breath in; or your throat may close up, becoming sore and constricted due to the inability to speak your truth.

This reminds me of a client I had in one of my 28-day detoxes. Whenever I'd ask the group if any issues were coming up, everyone else would talk but her. Finally, at the end of the detox, I had the chance to sit with her alone. I was feeding her my favorite watermelon and watercress salad with white balsamic vinegar when I saw her wince. I asked her if she had experienced any physical or emotional issues during the cleanse, and she said she hadn't. When I asked why she seemed to be in pain, she casually replied, "Oh, I have mouth sores. They're almost like little ulcers."

I realize how difficult it is for people to have a sense of themselves, but this woman's problem was much deeper—it involved not speaking up for herself. With some detective work (and Louise Hay's trusty blue bible), I found that my client never spoke her truth to her husband's mother and sister, who continually stomped all over her. Well, it was no coincidence that Mother's Day was the following weekend and she was supposed to have them both over to her home. She was terrified about the abuse she was going to have to endure.

I gave the woman Chinese herbs to help alleviate the physical symptoms, but I warned her they would only work as a Band-Aid. The real work was on an emotional level: she had to face her fears, open her throat chakra, and tell both her mother-in-law and sister-in-law right where to go.

She called me after the weekend, delivering her progress report with a healthy laugh. "The good news is that the sores are now completely gone. The bad news is that my family will never speak to me again."

Speaking your truth is part of the healing process. Don't be hard on yourself if you can't express yourself as quickly as you'd like. Give yourself credit for acknowledging the connection between finding your voice and emotional and physical manifestations. And keep this in mind: it has been observed that long-term survivors of cancer are the ones who learned to pay attention to their feelings, validate them, and talk about them honestly.

Share the Health

I know that I've been emphasizing the *me, me, me* throughout the healing process. But in life, there's always a balance between taking care of yourself and sharing your light. There is nothing like alleviating your own pain by helping others.

When clients call me with a variety of maladies, it coincidentally seems as though I've already dealt with their specific issue on some level. Many healers agree that the ability to heal actually stems from being able to empathize with others who have experienced similar pain. So whenever people tell me, "Wow, you've been sick a lot," I reply, "I'm not sick—I'm doing research and development."

I've loved finding the remedies that have healed me so that I could then share these insights with others. I've been blessed with the ability to pass on natural healing protocols for mononucleosis, strep throat, chronic ear infections, irritable bowel syndrome, or flu to others; and they in turn share those remedies with their families, friends, and neighbors. It spreads like fairy dust as we all heal each other. That's so much better than gossip, don'tcha think?

You might not be in a place at this moment to even think of sharing anything. That's okay—honor yourself. There were plenty of times I only had enough energy left for my immediate family.

Interestingly enough, my initiation to "sharing the health" began when I started to heal my family. Since the births of my children, I've strengthened them naturally. They are now teenagers, and neither of them has ever taken antibiotics. Raising them in the natural way has helped me become more confident, not only in healing myself, but also in sharing my guidance with others.

When my daughter, Paris, was six weeks old and had a cold, I couldn't wait to try all the remedies I'd learned about over the years, but it was a bit scary as well. As you delve into the world of natural remedies, you're going to have moments when you doubt yourself. One of those moments came when my son, Jet, was about three. He became so sick with an upper-respiratory cold that my remedies didn't seem to be working; in fact, he was getting worse. I took him to my natural doctor who helped me look at the emotional factors involved, and Jet improved right away.

You will increasingly become more confident each time you successfully find a remedy or modality that works. Then when you're feeling more equipped, and coming from a place of strength, you can begin to share your vitality with others. Service takes us out of the egocentric world of our diagnosis and gives us gratitude for our progress.

Speaking of growth . . . look how far you've come! Acknowledge all that you have accomplished and learned. Be proud of yourself for stretching the boundaries of your mind, body, and spirit. It's time to pat yourself on the back and move on to the final chapter, which is all about looking forward to your bright future!

CHAPTER EIGHT

Looking Forward

Stemming from ancient primitive beliefs, the word *disaster* actually means "from the stars." As this guide has taught you, when catastrophe strikes, it is meant to awaken you. You now know how to empower yourself, use your voice, and surrender. The hard part is over . . . you've arrived. Take a breath of gratitude right now—you've come a long way, baby! I am proud of you, and you should be, too. Go ahead and digest all that you have learned and use it as a platform as you look ahead. Going back to *Monopoly*, it's like you've been given a "Get Out of Jail Free" card, and you have a lot to look forward to.

After my brain surgery, my daughter, Paris, wrote her favorite saying on yellow Post-it notes all over my office: "If you could talk yourself into dying, you could just as easily talk yourself into living." Take that quote with you on your journey as you continue to transform from the old you to the new and improved you. Take your power back and run with it. Never stop, and never give up. What lies ahead is an exciting adventure, so laugh, sing, and *have fun!*

Aha Moments

As I look back at the pieces of this gigantic puzzle that is my life, I know that one of my Aha moments came when I realized beyond a shadow of a doubt that all that has ever happened to me was predestined. And from the moment I slammed my breast in the car door to the botched lumpectomy, from the metastasis to the discovery of my self, I have been graced with an incredible metamorphosis.

Your Aha moment might not come a week after you've been diagnosed, and it may not come after a month or even a year. But sometime after all the dust has settled, you *will* have that flash where the question as to why you've been chosen to endure this path gets answered. You will see it—the unadulterated reason you needed to be jolted awake by this experience. Maybe it was so you can help others. Maybe it was so you can leave your job to pursue your true passion. Maybe it was so you can learn to forgive the person who has hurt you the most in this life, the one you thought you could never forgive.

This mind-set may not be available for you just yet. But when you hear yourself saying, "Oh, *that's* why I had to get cancer," you'll know you have reached your Aha moment. Here's a scary thought: what if you went your entire life sound asleep, never to experience the eye-opening, life-changing thrill such a moment brings with it?

As I once heard Steve Jobs, co-founder of Apple, say, "Sometimes you have to drop out to drop in." It seems that he didn't see the point of college and thought it was too expensive for his parents to send him. After dropping out, he ended up taking a calligraphy class for fun—not seeing that it had any "purpose," per se, at the time. But when Steve was designing the first Mac, he used what he learned from the class to ensure that it had beautiful typography. He found that the calligraphy course had been more instrumental in developing the computer than the classes he'd taken in college.

Steve was fired from Apple in 1985; but, again, he had an Aha moment when he realized that this had allowed him to start two other companies, including Pixar. It also gave him the opportunity to meet his wife. Of course, he returned to Apple and has been extremely successful. And now that he's been diagnosed with cancer, who knows what amazing thing *that* will lead to?

Like Steve Jobs, you are one of the lucky ones who gets to have the Aha moment. As I tell people who call me with a new diagnosis, "What, you think you're the only one? No, you're going to go on just like everyone else who was diagnosed before you." I tell them they get to go on a health-awakening journey, and not only for themselves— for their families, too.

Sometimes when we can enlighten others in a positive way, we allow them to receive the gift of an Aha moment from our experiences. I once met with a woman with breast cancer whose teenage daughter was in a wheelchair with multiple sclerosis. I knew immediately that the mother was not going to make it. Although the methods I taught her wouldn't help her survive, they'd help change her daughter. In this woman's death, she actually saved her daughter's life.

●○●

Typically, we try to avoid land mines in our lives, but sometimes they just can't be avoided. We must face the destruction and keep on going. It becomes like a spiritual dig through hell, which then leads to resurrection. Like Winston Churchill said, "When you're going through hell, keep on going." We may not like what we see at first, and we may not agree with it—but it is in our best interests to pay attention to the message it's giving us.

One of the most enlightening lessons I have learned is that we're all active participants in our destiny. I believe I needed the turmoil I'd gone through so that I could find true peace. Now when things aren't working out in my world—when I am creating chaos or get a new diagnosis—I ask myself, "Dena, why are you attracting this into your life?"

I had an Aha moment when I discovered that so many challenges had presented themselves to me so I could connect with the light. I felt that God wouldn't give me more than I could handle, that somehow all of my challenges weren't meant to hurt me, but to awaken me. As I used to tell my dad, "We are here to learn our lessons, and every time we learn something huge, we move up a level until we graduate."

Many of us look only for pleasant experiences and try to avoid painful ones at all costs. I believe in using pain to catapult us to growth. To truly flow with life, the trick is nonattachment, nonresistance, and nonjudgment. Sri Nisargadatta Maharaj says it perfectly in I Am That: "Between the banks of pain and pleasure the river of life flows. It is only when the mind refuses to flow with life, and gets stuck at the banks, that it becomes a problem."

My favorite story is about a father and son who were living on a farm. One day a wild horse ran up to the farm, and all the neighbors said, "How lucky!" The father simply replied, "Maybe." The next day, the horse bucked the son off, causing him to break his leg. The neighbors all cried, "How unlucky!" The father again just replied, "Maybe." The next day, the troops arrived to recruit all the young men in the area for war, but the son couldn't go due to his newly broken leg. Again, the neighbors said, "How lucky." And again, the father replied, "Maybe."

The moral of the story is that we never know why something shows up in our lives until we have our Aha moments. We must let go of all outcomes and look forward to those moments arriving, and then embrace them when they appear.

New Beginnings

Happiness doesn't come from chasing what you don't have—it comes from appreciating what you *do* have. So be thankful for your body's way of speaking to you, teaching you, and working for you. Whether you have been diagnosed with cancer or any other challenge, look not to fight disease, but rather to create health. In other words, don't look at the deficit; instead, add up the infinite possibilities.

I never realized how blessed I really was until the day I met an older woman on my travels. She was in her 60s but looked about 110. She was hunched over, could barely walk, and had an oxygen tank attached to her. I asked her how she was, and she replied, "I'm okay, but they have been radiating me and chemotherapy-ing me for 15 years, and I'm lucky to be alive."

Was she, I wondered? Although I hadn't withered up like that through treatments (due to my wide array of healing tools), this picture scared the hell out of me. Right then and there, I decided that I was going to choose differently than this woman had.

For those of us who have endured testing, surgeries, chemotherapy, and radiation, we walk out of those hospital doors feeling like we've been set free when it's all over. Yet we will never be quite the same. Our wings may have been burned so we can't fly as high, and the fear will always remain somewhere in our subconscious—but the sun will shine brightly, carrying its message, not necessarily of hope (I never liked that word because I felt it was so weak and lacking). I discovered that confidence is the opposite of hope, and that is what we will walk through the doors of a new day with. No matter our destiny, we are now empowered with confidence in ourselves and all of our newfound knowledge.

When I started my journey a decade ago, doctors really didn't know what to tell a patient after they were done putting her through the wringer. Now, fortunately, more and more hospitals are implementing alternative-health-care initiatives and can direct you somewhere for support. There are also many targeted drugs on the horizon; as well as new forms of medical testing, procedures, and protocols to make your experience less dramatic and painful. These cutting-edge modalities will be less invasive and less toxic.

Today, we can look at this disease differently than ever before. We now live with many types of cancers, just as individuals do with diabetes. And we choose to not only survive, but to *kick ass*.

The Adventures of Death and Dying

When I decided to write this segment, some people said, "It's too negative." Well, I have faced the possibility of death myself—and I feel that it's not only a huge help to talk about it, but a ridiculous shame to hide from it. I don't want to tiptoe around this sensitive subject; rather, I prefer to bravely look at the infinite possibilities that death offers.

I love the way Pema Chödrön sums it up in one of my favorite books, *When Things Fall Apart*. She shares the idea that although death is a part of our everyday lives and is necessary, as we see it in the ending of the day, the change of seasons, the exhale of our breath, and the ending of relationships—we are still a culture that feels the need to hide from death. The bottom line is that fear of death is the reason for all of our suffering. Pema's answer is to move closer to that which we fear the most. Look right at it! Don't run from it.

Don't we all know that everyone will, at some time and in some way, die? The good news is that there are positive aspects of death and that it can be an exciting adventure. Let's take the mystery out of it as we look at all of its facets.

There are emotional deaths, which eradicate the old and give birth to the new (which we've learned all about in this book). There are spiritual deaths, in which we disconnect from a particular belief system. Then there are physical deaths, in which we transform our bodily selves, shedding our actual human form—or, as I like to call it, our vehicle. In this instance, we leave the earthly realm and move on to another life experience, or simply into the conscious realm of universal light.

Once we get over the fear of dying, we can really begin to live. I know about this firsthand. You see, I used to routinely be gripped by that fear, but this all changed when my brother died. Bradley and I were deeply connected in this incarnation; only 20 months apart, we came into this life as soul mates and teachers for one another. In his death, he taught me the most important lesson—and gave me the greatest gift—of all.

A few days after his death, he communicated to me through a dream: We were in an apartment, and he was packing, preparing to leave. I was begging him to stay, and he offered to take me with him. We went on a motorcycle ride up the side of a mountain, ever higher, feeling all-consuming joy, nothing that I'd ever felt in this life. As we came to the top, I saw an enormous pair of gates through the thickness of clouds, along with a man whom I recognized as a familiar spirit. My brother pleaded to the man for my entry, but with a calming smile, he shook his head no.

The gates opened, and my brother kissed and held me tight, just like he had the last time we'd seen each other in this life. As I watched him walk through the gates, I caught a glimpse of the sky there—it was like an aurora borealis, ablaze in pink, orange, and purple. Mansions lined the streets, and giant trees in full bloom with lotus blossoms dangling from them were everywhere. It truly did seem like a paradise.

I learned many things that night. For example, unlike our physical world—which is more about what we can touch, see, and hear—the higher realms seemed to be focused on what we could *feel,* as we're able to simply absorb the beauty and truth of everything.

When I woke up, the top of my head felt painful to the touch. It seemed entirely possible that I'd left my body through the crown of my head in order to learn about life after death. Yet I questioned the experience . . . until I came across books that described what I was so blessed to feel, including *Autobiography of a Yogi* by Paramahansa

Yogananda; *The Tibetan Book of Living and Dying,* by Sogyal Rinpoche; and *Life After Life,* by Raymond Moody, to name just a few.

After that dream I looked at my old compatriot, the fear of death, as it stubbornly stood its ground, not wanting to leave my side. I confronted it by asking, "What are you gonna do? Kill me if you like; take me now. If you're not going to, then begone with you." I saw this fear dissolve that very day. What we resist persists, and what we run away from will always chase us. Death was chasing me, but I stopped running. I chose to enjoy the adventure of my life, no matter where it took me.

If you have a fear of death, try this meditation:

> *Bringing in the white light through the top of your head, envision all-consuming fear and what it feels like in your stomach, head, throat, and heart. Tense up as you remember all the reasons you're afraid. Then ask the fear, "What can you really do to me?" Render it powerless as you face it, defy it, and laugh at it.*

We bring to us that which we're afraid of. My advice is to work on letting go of your fears, as they will only harm you. In fact, I have heard from reliable sources that when we die, we take with us the obsessive emotional drama and baggage of our lifetime. The goal is to rid ourselves of the excess crap so that our suitcase will be lighter for travel.

Eckhart Tolle, a spiritual guide to many, speaks of death in such a way that you don't just hear what he's saying—you somehow *know* it, as if you're remembering something you had forgotten long ago. His explanation is that death in itself does not really exist, and that this life is all an illusion. Wrap your brain around that one. Tolle relates the complexities of this subject by summing up an important source of spiritual writing from a book called *A Course in Miracles,* which states: "Nothing real can be threatened. Nothing unreal exists."

Tolle feels that the first exercise from this book says it all. You begin by looking at everyday objects around you, including your own body parts, and you simply remove yourself from all emotional attachment or value to those items by saying, "This table doesn't mean anything," "This arm doesn't mean anything," and so on. The weird thing is, as a young girl I would focus on certain objects and say their names over and over until they were meaningless, and the objects would dissolve. Try it now yourself. (But be patient, as it takes some time to grasp these concepts.)

Many scholars have suggested that you have two choices in physical death: (1) you will either take a new form so that you may learn further lessons in another life; or (2) if you are finished learning your lessons, you get to graduate from this illusion or Earth plane and receive the gift of being able to shed your form and go naked, so to speak. Ah, how freeing to be unencumbered by the physical form, which carries with it stress, intense emotions, and disease. The eternal "you" cannot be threatened or touched. And, as a parting gift, you get to take your spirit with you because your soul lives on forever and remembers all the lessons you have ever learned.

Now, I am acutely aware that it is much easier to digest these ideas when it comes to adults. It's the children that make it so much tougher. Whether you're trying to help them understand the passing of a parent or the loss of a friend, it can be very difficult for kids to accept death. From the perspective of a parent, I've explained such concepts to my children, preparing them for the possibility that one day they may lose my physical form. But I've let them know that I will be available in spirit for them, in the same way that my brother has always been there for me. Of course, they still will mourn the loss of my physical presence, but because of what I've shared with them, I'm sure they will be better equipped to handle the situation.

There doesn't seem to be any rhyme or reason when a child must leave this plane. This would be the most excruciating pain that exists, and I won't even begin to pretend that I know what it's like. I would endure all that I've been through a hundred more times just to prevent it from happening to my children. Yet cancer and death *do* happen to kids, and I feel that we must honor the lives and spirits of these special and wonderful souls who have so much to teach us and who live wondrous lives while they're here.

I recommend The Compassionate Friends, a support group for parents who have lost their children; along with books such as *After the Death of a Child: Living with Loss Through the Years,* by Ann K Finkbeiner. Both of these offer some ways to begin to move through such a devastating process.

Living in Remission

Living in remission can sometimes be like a scary movie where everyone else dies, and the final victim (you) is left alone to fight the scary monster. But it's as if you're simultaneously watching the movie and in it at the same time: There you are, sitting on the edge of your seat, cheering on the last survivor. As you watch in suspense, you're screaming, "Kill 'em, fight back harder, crush 'em, kick their ass!" (My kids hate watching movies with me, especially in a theater.)

Of course, the last victim standing always wins and triumphantly becomes the hero—but there is that moment before complete victory when the hero turns away from the monster, even though you're screaming. "No, don't turn away! Stab him one more time to make sure he's really dead!" But, of course, there's the hero turning away and dropping the weapon. You yell, "No, dummy, don't drop your weapon!" Sure enough, here comes the bloody enemy for a second round. Doesn't the hero know the evil beast must be stabbed in the heart with a silver sword and then have holy water thrown on him to seal his fate . . . ?

In this case, your weapons are good food, vitamins, healing modalities, spiritual remedies, emotional healing, and forgiveness. I have seen many clients forget that they're on a health-awakening journey, and they put down the weapons of their alternative-healing lifestyle—only to find themselves back in the ring with cancer once again. As you know, I myself had to be hit over the head a few times before I got it. If you stay focused and stay the course, victory will be yours.

Never forget, you must be your own advocate. Let your intuition lead the way so that you can create your very own bright and healthy future. Take all that you have learned and continue on the path of self-discovery as you find nourishing foods, alternative modalities, tinctures, remedies, supplements, and lifestyle therapies that work for you.

Accepting a situation doesn't mean accepting someone else's verdict about it. I love to show the doctors that they're wrong. It's the rebel in me. I've found that I am better off denying my diagnosis altogether and going about my healthy lifestyle without a worry or care.

I'd like to share a secret with you: We will all eventually leave this plane at some time in some way. It's up to us to decide when. We waste so much time and energy fighting everything in life. We need to stop now. Instead, we should spend our time and energy on healing, exploring our feelings, and repairing our relationships. As for me, I now absolutely laugh more, share more love, enjoy more sunrises and sunsets, appreciate each full moon, breathe in the smell of springtime, and delight in my children's voices.

While none of us knows what's in store for the future, I suggest that if you ever had a dream or a fear or a hidden passion, follow it, conquer it, go for it! Savor every second you have, but do the work you're here to do. When you surrender, you do not become inactive. On the contrary, you learn, build, strengthen, and—above all—kick ass.

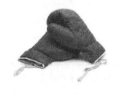

APPENDIX A

Final Checklist

I'd like to sum up the information you found in this guide by giving you a final checklist:

- Write it all down.
- Ask for what you need.
- Think twice before you act once; that is, do your research before having any procedures.
- Follow your intuition.
- Eat seaweed.
- Eliminate dairy, wheat and gluten, refined sugars, processed foods, and poor-quality animal fats from your diet.
- For sugar substitutes, try brown-rice syrup, barley malt, agave nectar, and B-grade real maple syrup.

- Note that some essential fats that our bodies require can be found in coconut milk and oil; unsweetened hemp milk, almond milk, and rice milk; avocados and avocado oil; seeds and nuts; high-quality olive oil; and sesame, coconut, flax, borage, and pumpkin-seed oils.

- Aspire to be more alkaline than acidic.

- Understand that grass-fed beef will leave your body with higher alkalinity levels.

- Avoid "angry" beef and chicken that have been pumped full of hormones and antibiotics.

- Don't eat food that has been left over for more than two days.

- Eighty percent of your diet should consist of fresh vegetables (and small amounts of seasonal fruit if you're in remission). Seventy percent of your diet may come from cooked food, including beans, legumes, grains, fish, and greens, with some sea vegetables. The rest can be in fresh vegetable juices (you may have a bit more if you live in a warm climate). Keep in mind that fresh-pressed vegetable juices provide nutrient-dense enzymes that are easily absorbed.

- Consume whole grains.

- Note that meat protein is difficult to digest. Also, meat remaining in the intestines becomes putrefied and leads to toxic buildup.

- Certain supplements allow the immune system to enable the body's own killer cells to destroy cancer cells. Such supplements include antioxidants like vitamins C, D, and the Bs; minerals; essential fatty acids; and several varieties made by Metagenics, such as Ultra Flora IB, Ultra Flora Plus, and Ultra Flora Plus DF. Vitamin E in particular is very important because it can promote programmed cell death (apoptotic activity) against a wide range of cancer-cell types, without damaging normal cells.

- Keep in mind that cancer cells don't thrive in an oxygenated environment. Exercising daily, deep breathing, and yoga all help you bring in more oxygen on a cellular level.

- Get moving: swim, dance, practice yoga or tai chi, run, walk . . . even crawl.

- *Poop!* Eliminate every single day—fake it till you make it, if you have to, with home enemas.

- Be in bed by 9:30 P.M., and asleep by 10:00 P.M.

- Reduce exposure to environmental toxins such as tap water, electromagnetic fields (EMFs), cleaning supplies, chlorine, and pollution.

- Meditate/pray regularly.

- Remember that cancer is a disease of the mind, body, and spirit. A positive spirit is imperative!

- Anger, resentment, and bitterness are toxic. Open your throat and heart chakra and speak your truth. Let it all hang out.

- Relax and enjoy life—and, above all, love and forgive yourself and others.

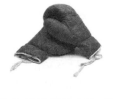

APPENDIX B

Remedies, Resources, and Readings

The next several pages are devoted to the resources I used throughout my health-awakening journey. Here you'll find the remedies that strengthened me, the healers who helped me, and the books and other readings that informed and guided me.

Remedies

Remedies for Surgery

— Consume the following drink 2–3 times per day for the first 2 days after surgery, then 1–2 times per day for the next week until you have fully rehydrated and regained your strength. (You can also continue this drink throughout radiation and chemotherapy.) Start with a fresh glass of filtered water and add these ingredients:

Organic pure cranberry concentrate juice, with no sugar added. This will support the kidneys and bladder while also aiding in pooping. Use 2 to 4 oz. in a large glass of water.

Milk thistle and dandelion root tincture help support healthy liver function. As an antioxidant, silymarin (the active agent in milk thistle) offers high protection against liver and cellular damage. Silymarin enhances the activity of white blood cells and works to protect against alcohol- or drug-induced liver damage as well as other liver damage. Use 1 dropper.

— **Pleurisy root tincture** is used to reduce swelling in lungs and release mucus from the lungs to ease cough and congestion. Use after surgery, which can cause deep congestion (this is what I did).

— **Endura** (from Metagenics) is an "energy and re-hydration formula" with added minerals and vitamins that will help boost your energy and rehydrate you. As the company explains: "Endura is a patented rehydration drink mix with a unique blend of electrolyte minerals that are found in muscle cells. It provides carbohydrates in the form of glucose polymers and fructose that are delivered in a special, balanced blend. It also delivers key electrolytes to replace those excreted through sweat during exercise, activity, and/or other dehydrating conditions. It provides high concentrations of absorbable magnesium, a mineral essential for cellular energy metabolism and glucose homeostasis." Use ½–1 scoop in a tall glass of water.

— **Ultra Potent-C** (from Metagenics) is a buffered delivery system designed to help prevent the stomach upset that is sometimes associated with high vitamin C intake. Ultra Potent-C Powder supports immune function by helping promote NK (natural killer) cell and white blood cell activity. Preliminary scientific research suggests that vitamin C in the form of Ultra Potent-C may result in improved uptake of the vitamin by white blood cells when compared to regular ascorbic acid. Use 1 scoop.

— **Chlorophyll** is a liquid green complex that's usually extracted from premium alfalfa leaves. It helps aid in elimination; in addition, it can cut down on digestive-tract odors that may result from a colostomy or ileostomy, or on fecal odor from incontinence. You may not be able to digest greens, so this is a great alternative right after surgery. (For long-term use, however, do not replace green vegetables with this liquid.) Use 1 or 2 Tbsp.

— Another great pre- and postsurgery drink is made with **Ultra Flora Plus DF** (from Metagenics). As the company explains, it is a "patented probiotic formula blended with a nondairy powder that provides highly viable, pure strains of *Lactobacillus acidophilus* and *Bifidobacterium lactis*, along with supportive factors" that build the good bacteria in your intestinal tract after drugs and antibiotics have assaulted the digestive tract and depleted the good bacteria. Take 1 tsp. in the A.M. and one in the P.M. on an empty stomach, dissolved in a small glass of water.

— **Scargo** (made by Home Health, and found in health-food stores such as Whole Foods) can be used topically to eliminate scars. My own scars faded to almost nothing after I used this product.

Remedies for Trauma and Shock

The following liquid tinctures can be used after surgery, radiation, or chemotherapy to reduce the stress of trauma and shock:

— **Traumeel liquid** (5–10 drops) can be taken without food or drink 3–4 times per day, for 2–3 days after surgery. Hold the liquid under your tongue for a few seconds, then swallow.

— **Arnica pellets** (a typical dose is 30 c, 4–5 pellets, held under the tongue with no food or water until they melt). Take this 4 times per day throughout the day for the first 2 days after surgery.

— **Bach Rescue Remedy** can be used the same way you used the liquid Traumeel, at the same dose.

Remedies for Radiation Therapy

For burning of the stomach and esophagus, start with a fresh glass of filtered water and add one or both of the following:

— **Aloe vera** is great for alleviating burning of the esophageal lining, stomach, or digestive tract due to radiation therapy. Use 2–4 Tbsp. of liquid aloe in a large glass of water.

— **Glutagenics** (from Metagenics) is another great option. This powder contains glutamine, licorice-root extract, and aloe-leaf extract. Use 1–2 heaping Tbsp. of this soothing powder in the water.

●○●

The items below are to be taken orally. They are homeopathic remedies that must be taken with no food or drink for at least 20 minutes before and after—and don't use any mint toothpaste, as mint cancels the effects of homeopathic remedies:

— **Traumeel liquid** (5–10 drops) can be taken without food or drink 3–4 times per day for 2–3 days after surgery. Hold the liquid under your tongue for a few seconds, then swallow.

— **Arnica pellets** (a typical dose is 30 c, 4–5 pellets, held under the tongue with no food or water until they melt). Take this 4 times per day throughout the day for the first 2 days after surgery.

— **Bach Rescue Remedy** can be used the same way you used the liquid Traumeel, at the same dose.

— **Detoxosode radiation liquid** should be taken at the dose of 1 capful under the tongue, twice per day, to rid the body of radiation toxicity. This liquid can be taken every day while going through radiation therapy.

Remedies for Chemotherapy

You may consume the hydrating aloe drink from the radiation section—have it 1–3 times per day as needed throughout chemotherapy. You may also add one or more of the powders below to the drink:

— **Glutagenics** (from Metagenics) supports a healthy intestinal lining, which is essential for healthy digestion, immune function, and liver function. It supports the integrity and immunity of a healthy intestinal lining. This is imperative while going through chemotherapy! This powder is a great formula for burning of the esophageal lining, which can happen during chemo and radiation therapies.

— **Cordyceps PS** (from Health Concerns) improves lung function, helps detoxify drugs from chemotherapy and radiotherapy, and boosts the immune system throughout these treatments.

— Oil derived from the aromatic herb **spikenard** helps elevate low blood pressure, which can result from the dehydration that chemotherapy can cause.

— **Coriolus PS** (from Health Concerns) is a medicinal-mushroom extract that Japanese researchers have shown possesses antitumor effects and stimulates the NK cells.

— **Marrow Plus** (from Health Concerns) can be taken for symptoms due to the suppression of bone-marrow functions caused by chemotherapy and radiation therapy. It helps offset the side effects from pharmaceuticals such as AZT, DHPG, antitumor agents, and other drugs that suppress white or red blood cells.

— **ImmuCore** (from Metagenics) provides a "multiple mechanistic approach" to support healthy immune system function, which it does through enhancing activities of macrophages, NK cells, and T cell subsets.

— **UltraInflamX Plus 360** (from Metagenics) is a powdered medical food that can be drunk as a shake or smoothie. It features selective "kinase response modulators," which have been shown to beneficially influence the function of enzymes that reduce the inflammation process. This product supplies a low-allergenic potential protein base in the form of rice protein, and is a potent antioxidant that may help improve overall health by reducing inflammation.

— **Proboulardi** (from Metagenics) has probiotic factors that are ideal for patients following any and all medical therapies that hinder the balance of intestinal microflora and healthy intestinal function. Chemotherapy and radiation, along with antibiotic or steroid use, hinder healthy microflora growth.

— **Liver Tone** (from Nature's Answer) contains milk thistle and dandelion root in a potent tincture. The liver is under duress while undergoing chemotherapy and radiation, so it's necessary to balance the enzymes there.

— **Chzyme** (from Health Concerns) includes a wide range of enzymes that help alleviate symptoms from chemotherapy and radiation, such as gas, bloating, cramping, regurgitation, nausea, and diarrhea. This great pill also works in treating nausea from motion sickness, hangovers, and the flu. It promotes absorption and digestion.

Remedies for General Use

— **Concentrated Liquid Fish Oil or EPA/DHA enteric-coated capsules** provide monounsaturated fatty acids that have been shown to fight inflammation.

— **Glycogenics** (from Metagenics) is an advanced, balanced B-complex formula that features 5-formyl tetrahydrofolate (calcium folinate), a special form of folic acid, for greater bioavailability. This new formula also delivers dramatically higher levels of vitamin B_{12} and is now vegetarian compatible. B vitamins are essential for normal growth and development, energy production, a healthy stress response, hormone balance, and homocysteine metabolism. Homocysteine is one of the key indicators of cardiovascular health and cognitive function.

— **UltraClear Plus pH** (from Metagenics) can be used as part of a cleanse, and it has added nutrients to enhance Phase II detoxification activity. It also promotes alkalization of urine.

— **E Complex-1:1** (from Metagenics) is a natural vitamin E supplement that features a 1:1 ratio of alpha-tocopherol to gamma-tocopherol. This ratio more closely resembles the tocopherol profile found naturally in vitamin E–rich plants, which is known for its antioxidant properties as well as its ability to regulate gene expression and signal healthy cells.

— **CoQ-10 ST** (from Metagenics) is an antioxidant that helps maintain heart, kidney, liver, and cellular health. The body uses coenzyme Q10 (or CoQ10) for cellular protection and growth. It also helps the immune system work better, makes the body better able to resist certain infections and types of cancer, and helps protect the heart from the damaging side effects of chemotherapy.

— **Oxygenics** (from Metagenics) is a blend of antioxidants and precursor nutrients that supports antioxidant systems within the body. It is a proprietary blend of beta-carotene and mixed carotenoids for balanced antioxidant protection, as well as milk thistle, quercetin, turmeric, and grape-seed extract. It helps protect against free radicals, which have been linked to many diseases.

— **Trancor** (from Metagenics) creates a beneficial balance between the effects of GABA and the excitatory effects of glutamate. Trancor was formulated to support a sense of tranquility in those who feel worried or nervous and is designed to work with the brain and central nervous system. I used it after brain surgery.

— **Bladder wrack** is made from a form of kelp that has been used medicinally for centuries, mainly because of its high iodine content. Tinctures of it stimulate thyroid function, are used in the relief of rheumatism and rheumatoid arthritis, and may be used both internally and as an external application for inflamed joints.

—**Turmeric and curcumin** have received much attention lately for their ability to combat human diseases such as cancer, inflammation, and atherosclerosis.

— **Vitamin D** maintains calcium balance, aids in cell differentiation, boosts immunity, has a role in insulin secretion and blood-pressure regulation, and helps fight cancer.

— **Calcium, magnesium, and potassium** relieve cramping through treatments.

— **Oregano oil** is antibacterial, antimicrobial, and antifungal. It aids in killing parasites. This works like tea-tree oil and grapefruit-seed extract all in one. Consider it an antibacterial herbal medicine that will kill microbes on contact. It is not a booster like echinacea, but a killer for acute inundation and protection when traveling. Use it for active infections, parasitic infections, *Candida albicans,* and molds.

— **Castor oil** can be used like this: spread it all over the liver region of the stomach, then place a flannel cloth on the liver for 20 minutes at night before bed to aid in elimination and the detoxification of the liver.

— **Licorice root,** in the form of root teas and chewable deglycyrrhizinated (or DGL) tablets, helps aid indigestion.

— **Vitamin infusions** are a mixture of sterile water with useful vitamins and minerals—such as vitamin C, magnesium, calcium, glutathione, and the vitamin B complex—administered intravenously. John Myers, M.D., was the first to develop vitamin and mineral IV infusions as part of a nutritional-repletion strategy for patients with chronic illness associated with nutritional depletion. His original mixture was nicknamed the "Myers cocktail."

Resources

Since the following list consists of people who helped me personally, most of them are located in or near Chicago, where I live. However, it would be good to contact them if you're looking for recommendations for practitioners in your own area. Here they are, in no particular order:

- Darek Zurawski—lymphatic drainage specialist and founder of Lymphatic Therapy Center. Contact: (847) 205-0211, or: **www.lymphatic-therapy.com.**

- Keith Berndtson, M.D.—performs vitamin infusions. Contact: (847) 232-9800.

- Darrell Brayboy, LAc—acupuncturist, shiatsu and Functional Medicine practitioner, founder of The Center for Preventive Medicine. Contact: (847) 242-0927.

- Pieter Van Heule, DC, DiHOM—holistic primary health-care provider with degrees in acupuncture, chiropractic, and homeopathy. Contact: (847) 251-0044.

- Shellea Swan, MS, LCPC, NCC—EMDR practitioner. Contact: (847) 226-0580.

- Razvan Rentea, M.D., and Andrea Rentea, M.D.—natural practitioners. Contact: (773) 583-7793.

- Thomas Pusateri, DC—chiropractor/applied kinesiology. Contact: (847) 934-4144.

- Zhengang Guo—Chinese herbalist and acupuncturist, founder of Life Rising and Ton Shen Health centers. Contact: (312) 842-2775, or: **www.liferising.com**.

- Dr. P. Sambhu—Ayurvedic practitioner. Contact: (847) 482-1488, or: **www.ayushya.com**.

- Merrick Ross, M.D.—professor of surgical oncology at MD Anderson Cancer Center. Contact: (877) MDA-6789, or: **www.mdanderson.org**.

- Douglas Merkel, M.D.—oncologist specializing in breast cancer. Contact: www.northshore.org.

- Malcolm M. Bilimoria M.D., FACS— oncologist; Director, Northwest Community Hospital's Illinois Center for Pancreatic and Hepatobiliary Diseases. Contact: (847) 483-9400, or: www.advancedsurgical.com.

- Ivan Ciric, M.D.—neurosurgeon. Contact: (847) 570-1440, or: www.northshore.org.

- Glenn J. Bubley, M.D.—oncologist; Director, Genitourinary Medical Oncology, Beth Israel Deaconess Medical Center; and Associate Professor, Department of Medicine, Harvard Medical School. Contact: (617) 667-2404, or: www.dfhcc.harvard.edu.

- Nicholas A. Vick, M.D.—neurologist. Contact: www.northshore.org.

- Max Vanorman—natural practitioner.

- Geoffrey Fenner, M.D.—plastic surgeon. Contact: (847) 716-2400, or: www.fennerplasticsurgery.com.

- Alyce Sorokie—colon therapist, founder of Partners in Wellness. Contact: (773) 868-4062, or: www.gutwisdom.com.

- Mary Farhi, M.D., MPH, NCMP—natural gynecologist. Contact: (847) 808-7070, or: www.cwcenter.yourmd.com.

Recommended Books

I seemingly devoured everything I could get my hands on that might assist me on my health-awakening journey. I don't mean to suggest that you need to read everything I did, but I thought you might appreciate seeing what has really helped me over the years with respect to my body, soul, and spirit. And rather than putting them all in one big ol' list, I categorized them into the following groups:

Inspirational

- *Autobiography of a Yogi,* by Paramahansa Yogananda
- *Bhagavad Gita: A New Translation,* by Stephen Mitchell
- *The Complete Collected Poems of Maya Angelou,* by Maya Angelou
- *Listen to the Warm,* by Rod McKuen
- *Mother Teresa: In My Own Words,* by Mother Teresa, compiled by José Luis González-Balado
- *Rumi: Bridge to the Soul,* by Coleman Barks
- *Thich Nhat Hahn: Essential Writings,* by Thich Nhat Hahn, edited by Robert Ellsberg
- *When Things Fall Apart: Heart Advice for Difficult Times,* by Pema Chödrön

Healing and Self-Help

- *Anatomy of the Spirit: The Seven Stages of Power and Healing,* by Caroline Myss

- *Anticancer: A New Way of Life,* by David Servan-Schreiber, M.D., Ph.D.

- *Between Heaven and Earth: A Guide to Chinese Medicine,* by Harriet Beinfield, LAc, and Efrem Korngold, LAc, OMD

- *Beyond Blame: A Full-Responsibility Approach to Life,* by Yehuda Berg

- *Change Your Thoughts, Change Your Life: Living the Wisdom of the Tao,* by Dr. Wayne W. Dyer

- *The Cure for All Cancers,* by Hulda Regehr Clark, Ph.D., N.D.

- *Dr. Max Gerson: Healing the Hopeless,* by Howard Strauss, with Barbara Marinacci

- *The Game of Life and How to Play It,* by Florence Scovel Shinn

- *Gut Wisdom: Understanding and Improving Your Digestive Health,* by Alyce M. Sorokie

- *Heal Your Body,* by Louise L. Hay

- *Knockout: Interviews with Doctors Who Are Curing Cancer—and How to Prevent Getting It in the First Place,* by Suzanne Somers

- *The Life You Were Born to Live: A Guide to Finding Your Life Purpose,* by Dan Millman

- *The Natural Remedy Book for Women,* by Diane Stein

- *The New York Times Guide to Alternative Health,* by Jane E. Brody, Denise Grady, and reporters of *The New York Times*

- *The Power of Intention: Learning to Co-create Your World Your Way,* by Dr. Wayne W. Dyer

- *The Power of Kindness: The Unexpected Benefits of Leading a Compassionate Life,* by Piero Ferrucci

- *Rainforest Remedies: One Hundred Healing Herbs of Belize,* by Rosita Arvigo, D.N., and Michael Balick, Ph.D.

- *Sacred Contracts: Awakening Your Divine Potential,* by Caroline Myss

- *The Secret,* by Rhonda Byrne

- *The 10 Best Questions for Surviving Breast Cancer: The Script You Need to Take Control of Your Health,* by Dede Bonner, Ph.D.

- *Timeless Healing: The Power and Biology of Belief,* by Herbert Benson, M.D.

- *Trust Your Vibes: Secret Tools for Six-Sensory Living,* by Sonia Choquette

- *Way of the Peaceful Warrior: A Book that Changes Lives,* by Dan Millman

Eye-Opening Commentary

- *The Emperor of All Maladies: A Biography of Cancer,* by Siddhartha Mukherjee

- *Fast Food Nation: The Dark Side of the All-American Meal,* by Eric Schlosser

- *Genetic Roulette: The Documented Health Risks of Genetically Engineered Foods,* by Jeffrey M. Smith

- *Organic Manifesto: How Organic Farming Can Heal Our Planet, Feed the World, and Keep Us Safe,* by Maria Rodale

- *Seeds of Deception: Exposing Industry and Government Lies About the Safety of the Genetically Engineered Foods You're Eating,* by Jeffrey M. Smith

- *Slaughterhouse: The Shocking Story of Greed, Neglect, and Inhumane Treatment Inside the U.S. Meat Industry,* by Gail A. Eisnitz

Exercise and Nutrition

- *The Cancer Prevention Diet: Michio Kushi's Macrobiotic Blueprint for the Prevention and Relief of Disease,* by Michio Kushi, with Alex Jack

- *A Consumer's Dictionary of Food Additives,* by Ruth Winter, MS

- *Eat Right 4 Your Type: The Individualized Diet Solution to Staying Healthy, Living Longer & Achieving Your Ideal Weight,* by Peter J. D'Adamo

- *Healthy Highways: The Traveler's Guide to Healthy Eating,* by Nikki and David Goldbeck

- *Medicine Within Our Bodies,* by James W. McNeil
- *Mindful Movements: Ten Exercises for Well-Being,* by Thich Nhat Hahn
- *Pocket Guide to Macrobiotics,* by Carl Ferré
- *Sugar Blues,* by William Dufty

Cookbooks

- *The Angelica Home Kitchen,* by Leslie McEachern
- *The Anti-Cancer Cookbook,* by Julia B. Greer, M.D., M.P.H.
- *The Candle Cafe Cookbook,* by Joy Pierson and Bart Potenza, with Barbara Scott-Goodman
- *Changing Seasons Macrobiotic Cookbook,* by Aveline Kushi and Wendy Esko
- *The Flavor Bible,* by Karen Page and Andrew Dornenburg
- *The Kripalu Cookbook: Gourmet Vegetarian Recipes,* by Atma Jo Ann Levitt
- The Moosewood Restaurant cookbook series, by the Moosewood Collective
- *New Vegetarian,* by Robin Asbell
- *The Taste for Living World Cookbook,* by Beth Ginsberg and Mike Milken
- *The Wellness Cookbook for a Healthy U,* by Dena Mendes (downloadable version available at my website)

Helpful Articles, Websites, and Blogs

Along with my own site, Dena's Healthy U (**www .denashealthyu.com**), I recommend the following:

- Baking Soda Treatment Method:
  www.curenaturalicancro.com

- Cafe Gratitude—collection of 100% organic
  vegan restaurants: **http://cafegratitude.com**

- Crazy Sexy Cancer—an inspirational site
  including a blog, documentary, and books
  about Kris Karr's journey with cancer:
  www.crazysexycancer.com

- Cure Today—a site providing a magazine,
  educational forums, and online tools for
  those diagnosed with cancer:
  http://curetoday.com

- EmpowHER—information on women's health
  and wellness: **www.empowher.com**

- Gavin Evanston—Chicago-based boutique
  with fantastic clothing and accessories:
  www.shopgavin.com

- Gayl Walder Wellness—site for the Healing in
  Motion DVD series: **www.gaylwalder.com**

- The Heart Beet—a "webazine" about holistic
  health and mind-body-spirit issues:
  www.theheartbeet.com

- Her Future—a social-networking site to
  connect girls and women with mentors:
  www.herfuture.com

- High Tech Health International—for information on their infrared sauna: **www.hightechhealth.com/html /sauna_main.htm**

- Imerman Angels—a service that connects cancer fighters, survivors, and caregivers: **www.imermanangels.org**

- Jai Lifestyle—products and services promoting wellness and fitness for athletes and ordinary people alike: **www.jai-lifestyle.com**

- Karyn's—website of raw-food chef Karyn Calabrese, with information on her restaurants, holistic day spa, and various services: **www.karynraw.com**

- "Kripalu Recipes"—a collection of recipes from the newsletter of the Kripalu Center for Yoga & Health: **www.kripalu.org/article/270**

- Kushi Institute—a macrobiotic educational center in Becket, MA: **www.kushiinstitute.org**

- Living Organic—a site for articles on organic food, clothing, and gardening: **www.living-organic.net**

- Livingreen—an online retailer of healthier, more sustainable household products and building materials: **www.livingreen.com**

- "Lymphatic Drainage Exercise"—on the RightHealth site: **www.righthealth.com /topic/Lymphatic_Drainage_Exercise**

- Merz Apothecary: www.merzapothecary.com

- 101 Cookbooks—a site featuring vegetarian-recipes and a blog focusing on natural, whole foods: www.101cookbooks.com

- The Raj, Maharishi Ayurveda Health Spa Resort: www.theraj.com

- "Sourcing Healthy, Grass-Fed Meats," by Laura Klein—on the Organic Authority site: www.organicauthority.com/organic-food /organic-food-articles/sourcing-healthy -grass-fed-meats.html

- SunFire Super Foods: http://sunfiresuperfoods.com

- "Toxic Household Chemical Facts and Statistics"—on the Best of Mother Earth blog: http://bestofmotherearth.com/2009/04 /28/toxic-household-chemical-facts-and -statistics

- TreeHugger—providing green and sustainability news: www.treehugger.com

- Walsh Natural Health: www.walshnaturalhealth.com

- Your Healthy Liver—website of self-proclaimed "Liverguru," Dee; contains information on how a healthy liver leads to a healthy life: www.liverguru.com

- Zema's Madhouse Foods, Inc.—creators of ancient-grain, gluten-free baking mixes: www.zemasmadhousefoods.com

●○●○●

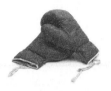

GRATITUDE

To my children, you are my true inspiration. I am eternally grateful for all that you teach me every single day. God gifted me with amazing children whom I adore. You are the loves of my life. Thank you for choosing me as your mom!

- To Jet, my sweet and sensitive boy, thank you for always making me laugh through even the most treacherous storms.

- To Paris, my sweet pumpkin-pie girl, for showing me how a loyal, loving, and meaningful friendship between two women can be, even when they are mother and daughter.

- To August and Brice, my sons from another mother, thank you for allowing me to be a part of your lives. I am so very proud of you both.

To Steven, thank you for all that you have taught me, for your support in so many ways through so many years, and the wonderful gifts you shared. I am forever grateful to you for our amazing children and loving them with me. You will always hold a loving place in my heart.

A special acknowledgment to my dear, sweet, always-missed brother, Bradley—thank you for watching over me every day. Not a day goes by that I don't think of you and miss you.

To my loving, supportive, and most generous grand-parents, thank you for being like parents to me.

To my amazing friends, you came each time I needed you most to help me heal. The list is long—you know who you are. Thank you for tirelessly sharing your love, support, and time unconditionally. I was so blessed that you all rallied together on my behalf during my health-awakening experiences. With all my love and gratitude, I thank those of you who shared.

To my most patient, generous friends who listened, read, and helped breathe life into this book: Betsy D'Alba, Claudia Lubin, Juli Jacobs, Michael Anderson, and Alison Liguori.

To Lance, your unwavering support, love, patience, and commitment have been lifesaving. I could never have done any of this without you. My deep love and gratitude for all space and time. Thank you for all that you have shared and taught me about myself.

To my family . . . thank you. You showed me how to be a more aware mother to my children. I bless all of you for showing me the truth and setting me free through forgiveness. God bless you, and I wish you all the best in your lives.

To my magical and gifted healers, each one of you came into my life at the perfect time when I needed you most. I bless you all, as you taught, gave, shared, and healed me on so many levels.

To the clients, neighbors, and families who have called on me, thank you for trusting me. You have given me the distinct privilege to share the health.

To my team of editors—Jill Kramer, Shannon Littrell, Eileen O'Halloran, and Jon VanZile—who made my words and experiences flow into a healing gift for all to read, the lessons have been invaluable. I bless you for your unlimited patience, constant support, and unwavering commitment.

David, I would like to especially thank you for your faith and generous support.

To the creative team who made it all look great—bless you for your patience! Photography: Lance Cutler; cover art: Jessica Rosengard; stylists: Lauren Cavallo Runzel from Gavin Evanston, and Mary from Ami Ami, Deerfield; creative consultant: Juli Jacobs; and Hay House creative director Christy Salinas.

Finally, I would like to thank Hay House for giving me the opportunity of a lifetime. To "share the health" with so many is truly my dream come true. God bless you for making it happen.

With respect, love, and gratitude,
Dena

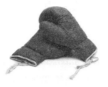

ABOUT THE AUTHOR

Dena Mendes, ND, is a well-respected public-health specialist and consultant. She is a cancer survivor who bravely combines alternative therapies to "kick cancer's ass." After numerous cancer-related surgeries and chemotherapy regimens, she's still kickin' ass. She is founder of the not-for-profit Pink Foundation—an organization whose mission is to educate people facing health challenges with alternative and holistic support.

Dena received her B.A. in communications/broadcast journalism from Arizona State University while also studying public health, has attended programs at Harvard and Northwestern universities, and holds a doctor of naturopathy degree. In addition, she is licensed and certified as a health coach, holistic yoga instructor, holistic chef, and pranic healer.

Dena is a motivational speaker who inspires audiences with her riveting and candid anecdotal stories. She empowers audiences to grow a new sense of themselves as she compassionately guides them through their own health-awakening journeys. She has developed "the Food Detectives," an educational program for K–12 schools, which encourages children to make wise nutritional choices. The Food Detectives have brought this essential program to hundreds of schools across the country, including Northwestern University.

Dena writes stories for children, such as "Princess Paris Pink," developed in 2000 to adorn a pink cow statue featured in front of FAO Schwarz for the "Cows on Parade" art event in Chicago, Illinois. "Princess Paris Pink" teaches kids about overcoming prejudice and learning acceptance. She also wrote and directed a rhythmic, surreal satire called *Standard of Care,* in which the audience joins her on a theatrical journey down the proverbial rabbit hole of cancer.

Dena lives with her two children near Chicago.

Website: **www.denashealthyu.com**

●○● WRITE IT DOWN! ●○●

●○● WRITE IT DOWN! ●○●

●○● WRITE IT DOWN! ●○●

●○● WRITE IT DOWN! ●○●

●○● WRITE IT DOWN! ●○●

●○● WRITE IT DOWN! ●○●

We hope you enjoyed this Hay House book. If you'd like to receive our online catalog featuring additional information on Hay House books and products, or if you'd like to find out more about the Hay Foundation, please contact:

Hay House, Inc., P.O. Box 5100, Carlsbad, CA 92018-5100
(760) 431-7695 or (800) 654-5126
(760) 431-6948 (fax) or (800) 650-5115 (fax)
www.hayhouse.com® • www.hayfoundation.org

●○●

Published and distributed in Australia by: Hay House Australia Pty. Ltd.,
18/36 Ralph St., Alexandria NSW 2015 • *Phone:* 612-9669-4299
Fax: 612-9669-4144 • www.hayhouse.com.au

Published and distributed in the United Kingdom by: Hay House UK, Ltd.,
292B Kensal Rd., London W10 5BE • *Phone:* 44-20-8962-1230
Fax: 44-20-8962-1239 • www.hayhouse.co.uk

Published and distributed in the Republic of South Africa by:
Hay House SA (Pty), Ltd., P.O. Box 990, Witkoppen 2068
Phone/Fax: 27-11-467-8904 • www.hayhouse.co.za

Published in India by: Hay House Publishers India, Muskaan Complex,
Plot No. 3, B-2, Vasant Kunj, New Delhi 110 070
Phone: 91-11-4176-1620 • *Fax:* 91-11-4176-1630 • www.hayhouse.co.in

Distributed in Canada by: Raincoast, 9050 Shaughnessy St.,
Vancouver, B.C. V6P 6E5 • *Phone:* (604) 323-7100
Fax: (604) 323-2600 • www.raincoast.com

●○●

<u>Take Your Soul on a Vacation</u>

Visit **www.HealYourLife.com®** to regroup,
recharge, and reconnect with your own magnificence.
Featuring blogs, mind-body-spirit news,
and life-changing wisdom from Louise Hay and friends.

Visit **www.HealYourLife.com** today!